ATLAS OF TUMORS OF THE SKIN

ALFRED W. KOPF, M.D.

Professor, Department of Dermatology,
New York University School of Medicine;
Head, Oncology Section, Skin and Cancer Unit,
University Hospital, New York University Medical Center

ROBERT S. BART, M.D.

Associate Professor, Department of Dermatology,
New York University School of Medicine;
Associate Head, Oncology Section, Skin and Cancer Unit,
University Hospital, New York University Medical Center

RAFAEL ANDRADE, M.D.

Professor and Chairman, Department of Dermatology,
La Salle Medical School, La Salle University of Mexico;
Consultant in Dermatology and Chief, Section of Dermatopathology,
Departments of Dermatology and Pathology,
General Hospital S.S.A. of Mexico City;
Formerly Associate Professor of Dermatology,
New York University School of Medicine,
and Director, Laboratory of Skin Pathology,
Skin and Cancer Unit, New York University Medical Center

1978

W.B. SAUNDERS COMPANY
Philadelphia London Toronto

W. B. Saunders Company: West Washington Square
Philadelphia, PA   19105

1 St. Anne's Road
Eastbourne, East Sussex BN21 3UN, England

1 Goldthorne Avenue
Toronto, Ontario M8Z 5T9, Canada

Library of Congress Cataloging in Publication Data

Kopf, Alfred W

Atlas of tumors of the skin.

Includes index.

1. Skin — Tumors — Atlases.   I. Bart, Robert S., joint author.
   II. Andrade, Rafael, joint author.   III. Title.

RC280.S5K66   616.9'92'770222   77–16978

ISBN 0–7216–5487–8

Atlas of Tumors of the Skin   ISBN   0-7216-5487-8

PREFACE

Since 1955 photographs have been taken of almost all patients who have come to the Oncology Section of the Skin and Cancer Unit, New York University Medical Center, for diagnosis and management of cutaneous tumors. All of these photographs, numbering approximately 45,000, were reviewed for this atlas. About 900 have been selected to depict most types of cutaneous tumors, both benign and malignant. In some instances, several variants of the same type of tumor are included; for example, we have selected many photographs of basal-cell carcinomas in order to emphasize the variability of clinical morphology of this very common type of skin cancer.

The photographs are arranged in alphabetical order. If you cannot find the photographs of a neoplasm in the atlas under the designation you normally use, we recommend that you check the index for cross references.

We have included the following information concerning each lesion, when available; sex, age at time of consultation, duration stated by patient, site of photographed lesion, and whether the diagnosis was histologically verified.

There is no other written material because we consider this atlas a companion volume to the comprehensive textbook *Cancer of the Skin* edited by Rafael Andrade, Stephen Gumport, George Popkin and Thomas Rees. This atlas presents many more photographs than would be possible to include in any standard text. A review of the photographs will demonstrate a panorama of most types of benign and malignant cutaneous neoplasms.

We are indebted to the staff of the Skin and Cancer Unit, New York University Medical Center for their continued cooperation, which made this atlas possible.

ALFRED W. KOPF, M.D.
ROBERT S. BART, M.D.
RAFAEL ANDRADE, M.D.

ACANTHOSIS NIGRICANS. Male; *age* 48 years; *duration* 3 months; axilla.

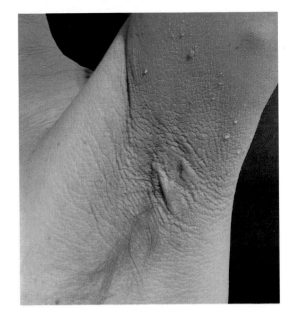

ACANTHOSIS NIGRICANS. Female; *age* 30 years; *duration* 1 year; nuchal area; confirmed by biopsy.

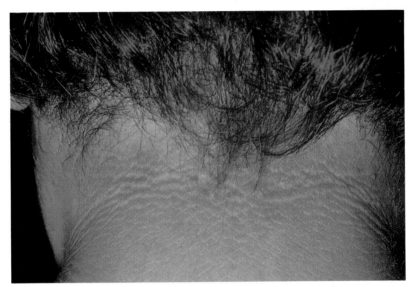

ACANTHOSIS NIGRICANS. Male; *age* 48 years; *duration* 3 months; nuchal area.

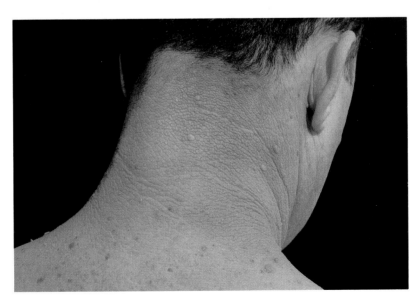

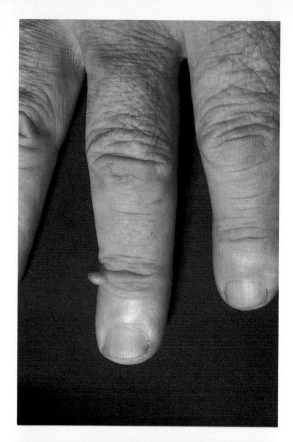

ACQUIRED DIGITAL FIBROKERATOMA. Male; *age* 68 years; *duration* 40 years; finger; confirmed by biopsy.

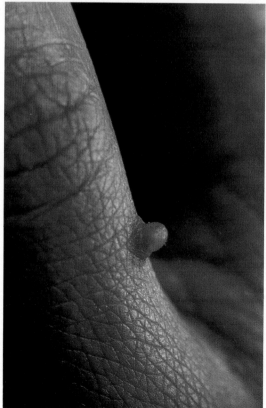

ACQUIRED DIGITAL FIBROKERATOMA. Male; *age* 54 years; *duration* 5 years; base of thumb; confirmed by biopsy.

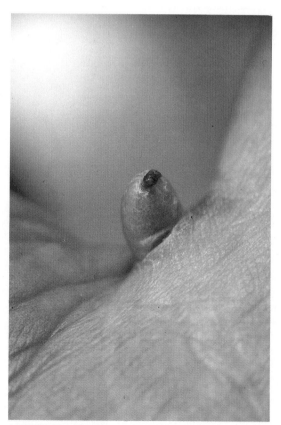

ACQUIRED DIGITAL FIBROKERATOMA. Female; *age* 13 years; *duration* 3 years; thumb; confirmed by biopsy.

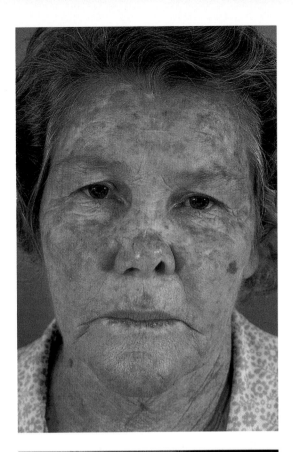

ACTINIC KERATOSES. Female; *age* 65 years; *duration* 20 years; face (especially forehead, nose and cheeks).

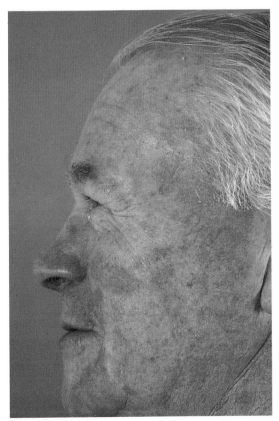

ACTINIC KERATOSES. Male; *age* 64 years; *duration* several years; cheek; confirmed by biopsy.

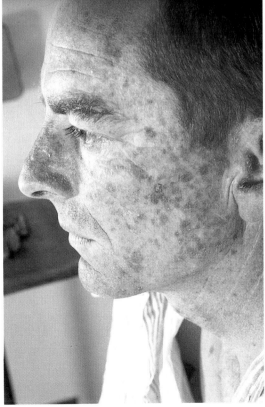

ACTINIC KERATOSES. Male; *age* 38 years; *duration* several years; face; confirmed by biopsy.

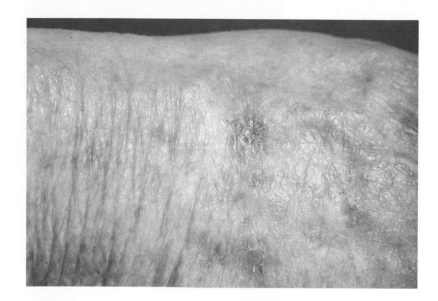

ACTINIC KERATOSES. Female; *age* 74 years; dorsum of hand; confirmed by biopsy.

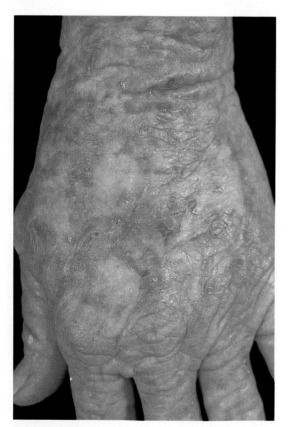

ACTINIC KERATOSES. Female; *age* 65 years; *duration* 20 years; hand.

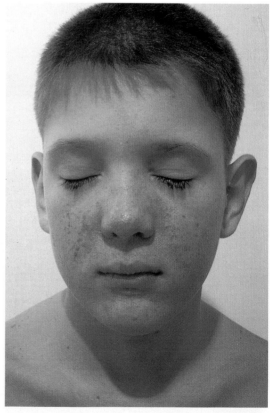

ADENOMA SEBACEUM. Male; *age* 13 years; *duration* since early childhood; face; confirmed by biopsy.

ADENOMA SEBACEUM. Female; *age* 15 years; *duration* many years; face.

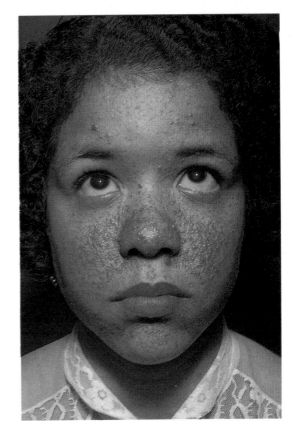

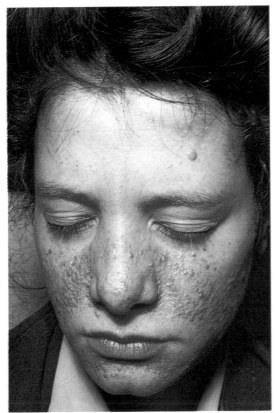

ADENOMA SEBACEUM. Female; *age* 17 years; *duration* 15 years; face.

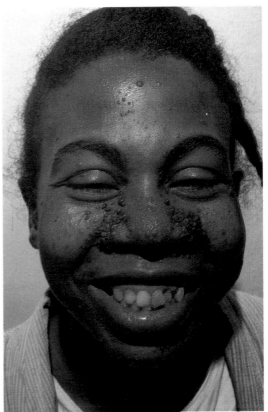

ADENOMA SEBACEUM. Female; *age* 13 years; face.

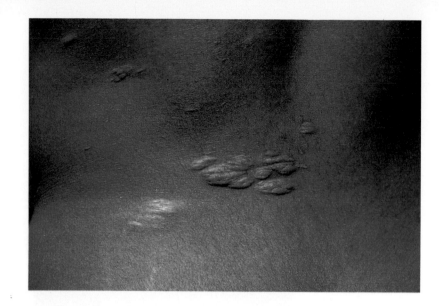

ADENOMA SEBACEUM (SHA-GREEN PLAQUES). Female; lumbrosacral area.

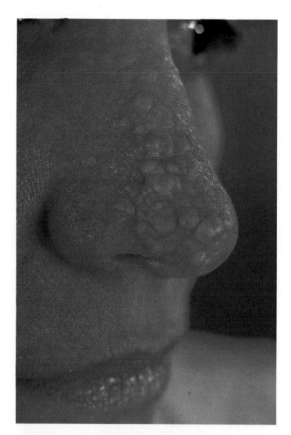

ADENOMA SEBACEUM. Female; *age* 38 years; *duration* 21 years; nose; confirmed by biopsy.

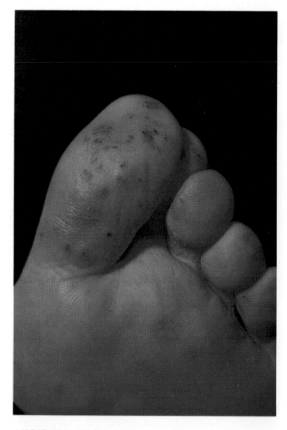

ANGIOKERATOMA (MIBELLI). Female; *age* 15 years; *duration* 9 years; foot.

ANGIOKERATOMA (MIBELLI). Female; *age* 15 years; *duration* 9 years; foot.

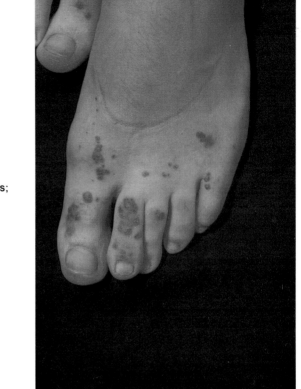

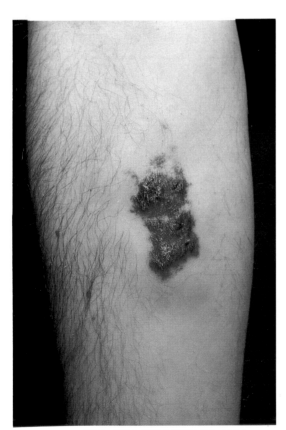

ANGIOKERATOMA (CIRCUMSCRIPTUM). Male; *age* 22 years; *duration* since birth; forearm; confirmed by biopsy.

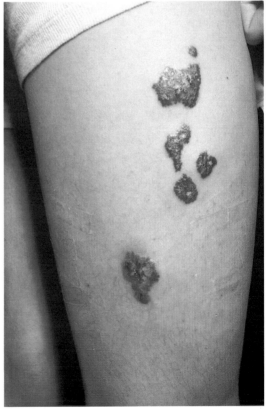

ANGIOKERATOMA (CIRCUMSCRIPTUM). Male; *age* 17 years; *duration* 1 year; thigh; confirmed by biopsy.

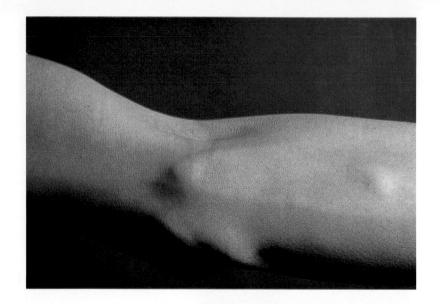

ANGIOLIPOMAS Male; *age* 55 years; *duration* 3 years; upper extremity; confirmed by biopsy.

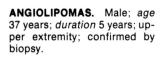

ANGIOLIPOMAS. Male; *age* 37 years; *duration* 5 years; upper extremity; confirmed by biopsy.

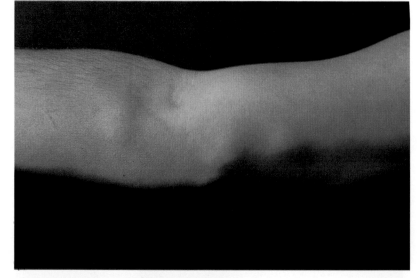

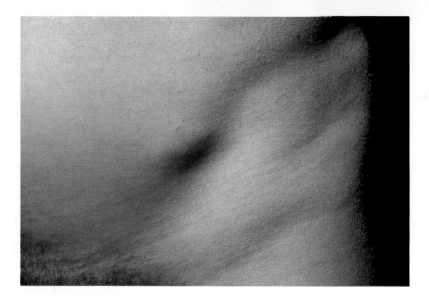

ANGIOLIPOMA. Male; lower abdomen.

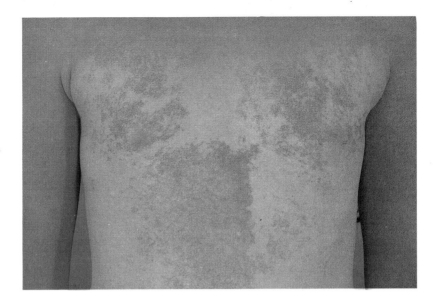

ANGIOMA SERPIGINOSUM.
Male; trunk.

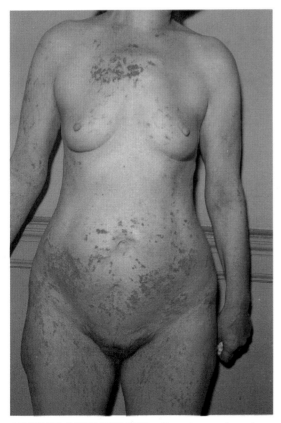

ANGIOMA SERPIGINOSUM. Female; trunk and extremities.

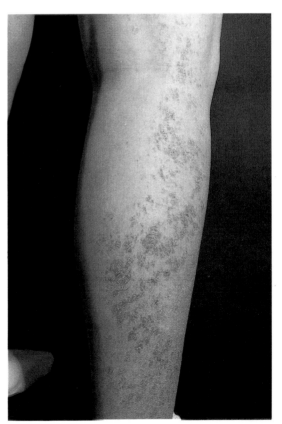

ANGIOMA SERPIGINOSUM. Male; *age* 12 years; *duration* since birth; lower extremity; confirmed by biopsy.

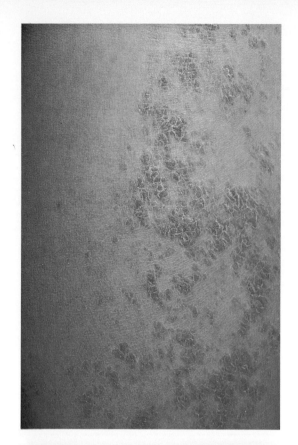

ANGIOMA SERPIGINOSUM. Male; *age* 12 years; *duration* since birth; leg; confirmed by biopsy.

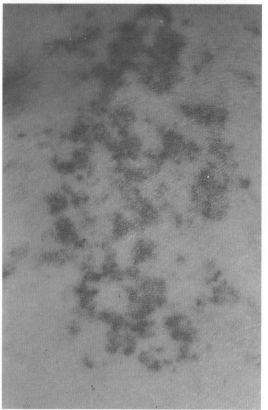

ANGIOMA SERPIGINOSUM. Female; back.

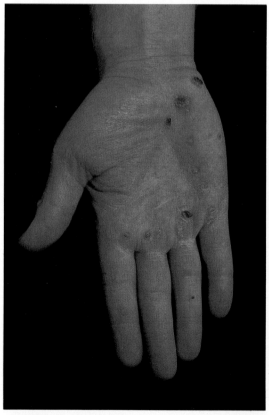

ARSENICAL KERATOSES. Male; *age* 40 years; hand; confirmed by biopsy.

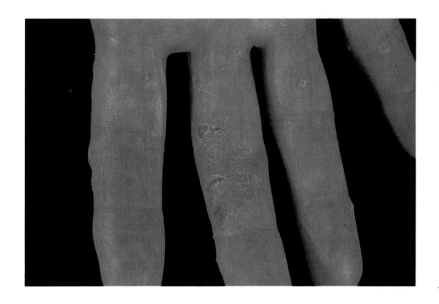

ARSENICAL KERATOSES.
Female; *age* 72 years; *duration* many years; palm.

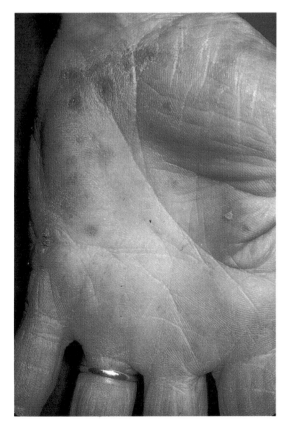

ARSENICAL KERATOSES. Male; *age* 77 years; *duration* 25 years; palm.

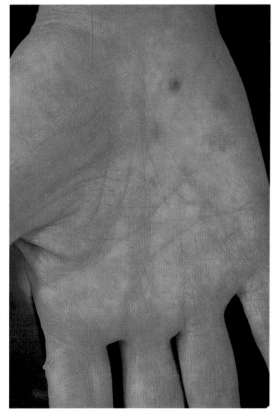

ARSENICAL KERATOSES. Female; *age* 72 years; *duration* many years; fingers.

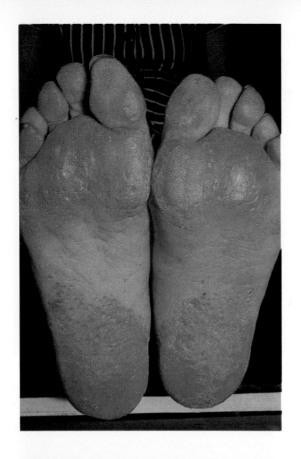

ARSENICAL KERATOSES. Female; *age* 41 years; *duration* 15 years; soles.

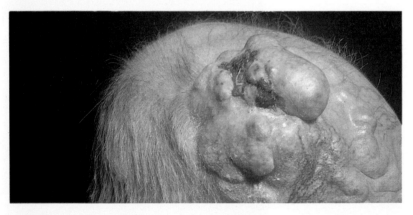

ARTERIOVENOUS FISTULA. Male; *age* 78 years; *duration* 50 years; scalp.

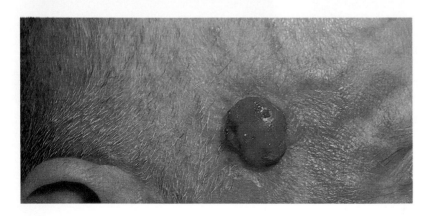

ATYPICAL FIBROXANTH- OMA. Male; *age* 82 years; *duration* 1 month; confirmed by biopsy.

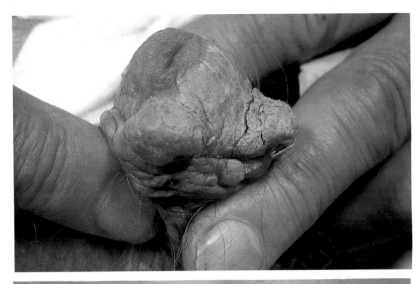

**BALANITIS, PSEUDOEPI-
THELIOMATOUS KERATOTIC
AND MICACEOUS.** Male; *age*
80 years; *duration* 3 years;
penis; confirmed by biopsy
(cutaneous horn with pseudo-
epitheliomatous hyperplasia).

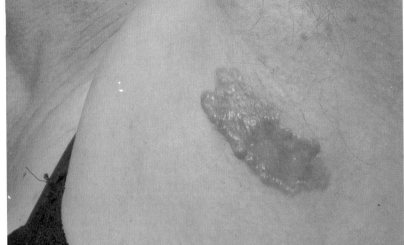

BASAL-CELL CARCINOMA.
Female; *age* 60 years; *duration* 35 years; axilla; confirmed
by biopsy.

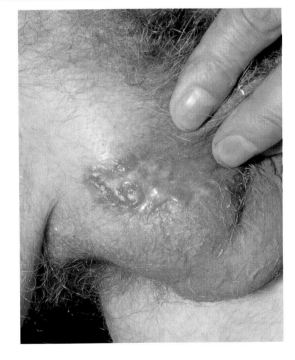

BASAL-CELL CARCINOMA. Male; *age* 71 years;
duration 6 years; scrotum; confirmed by biopsy.

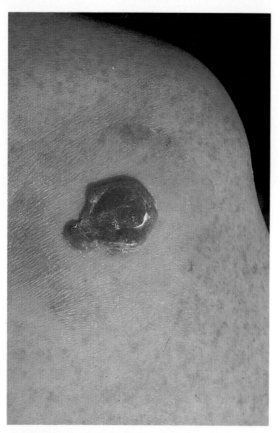

BASAL-CELL CARCINOMA. Female; *age* 69 years; *duration* 2 years; posterior aspect of shoulder; confirmed by biopsy.

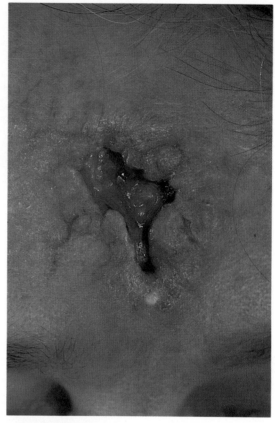

BASAL-CELL CARCINOMA. Female; *age* 53 years; *duration* 5 years; forehead; confirmed by biopsy.

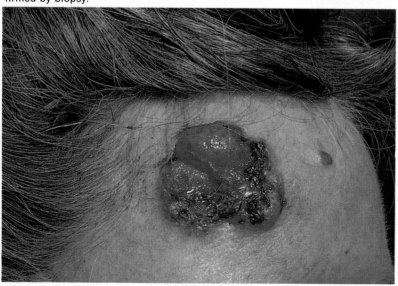

BASAL-CELL CARCINOMA. Female; *age* 64 years; *duration* 2 years; forehead; confirmed by biopsy.

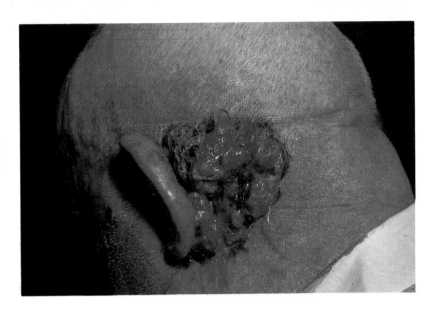

BASAL-CELL CARCINOMA.
Male; *age* 80 years; retroauricular area; confirmed by biopsy.

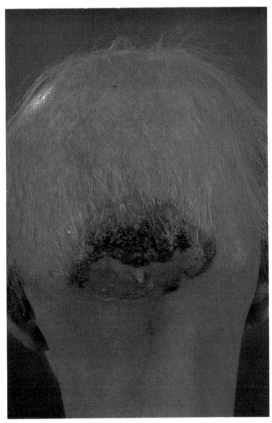

BASAL-CELL CARCINOMA. Female; *age* 57 years; *duration* 10 years; occipital area; confirmed by biopsy.

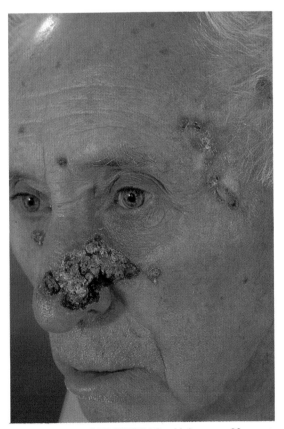

BASAL-CELL CARCINOMAS. Male; *age* 80 years; *duration* 5 years; face; confirmed by biopsy.

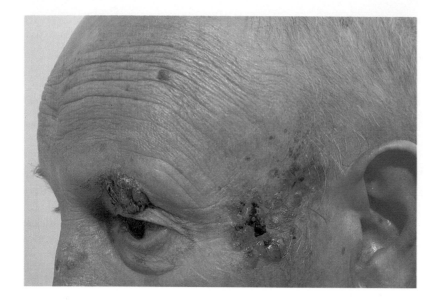

BASAL-CELL CARCINOMAS.
Male; *age* 71 years; *duration* 4 years; temple, eyelid, nose; confirmed by biopsy.

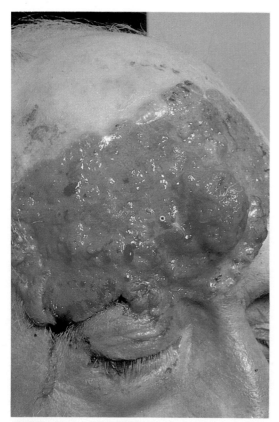

BASAL-CELL CARCINOMA. Male; *age* 82 years; forehead, eyebrow; confirmed by biopsy.

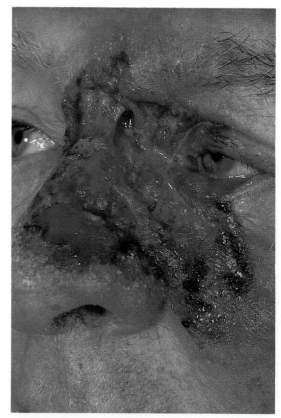

BASAL-CELL CARCINOMA. Male; *age* 62 years; *duration* 17 years; nose, eyelids, cheek; confirmed by biopsy.

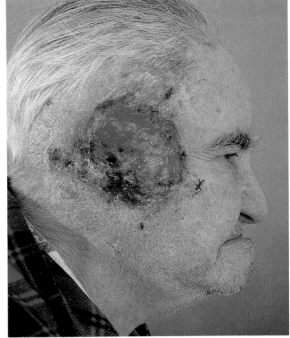

BASAL-CELL CARCINOMA. Male; ear.

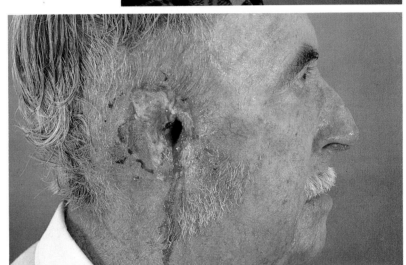

BASAL-CELL CARCINOMA.
Male; ear.

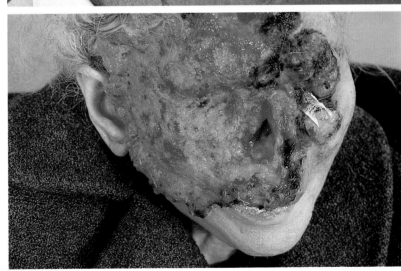

BASAL-CELL CARCINOMA.
Female; face.

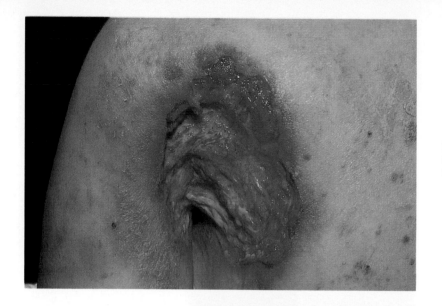

BASAL-CELL CARCINOMA.
Female; *age* 71 years; *duration* 14 years; axillary area; confirmed by biopsy.

BASAL-CELL CARCINOMA.
Male; *age* 63 years; *duration* 13 months; forearm; confirmed by biopsy.

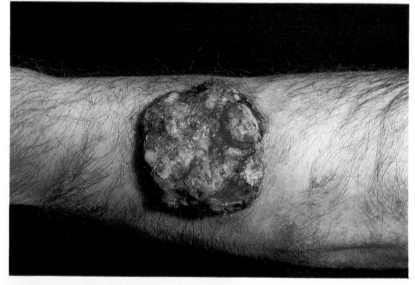

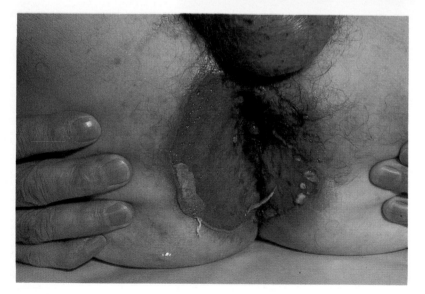

BASAL-CELL CARCINOMA.
Male; *age* 70 years; *duration* 3 years; perianal; confirmed by biopsy.

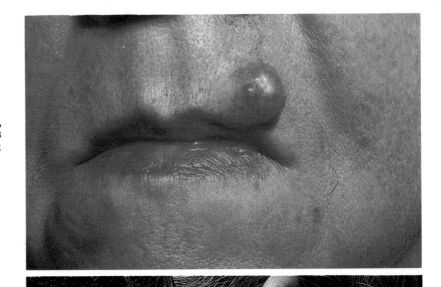

BASAL-CELL CARCINOMA, CYSTIC. Female; *age* 63 years; *duration* 5 years; lip; confirmed by biopsy.

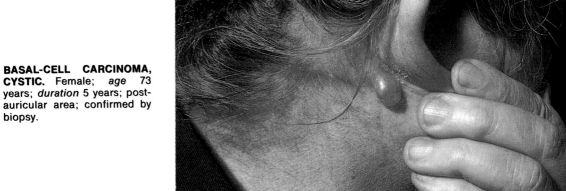

BASAL-CELL CARCINOMA, CYSTIC. Female; *age* 73 years; *duration* 5 years; post-auricular area; confirmed by biopsy.

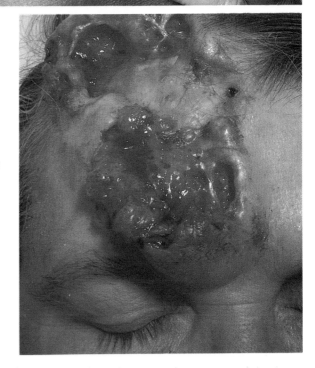

BASAL-CELL CARCINOMA, EXTENSIVE. Female; *age* 42 years; forehead; confirmed by biopsy.

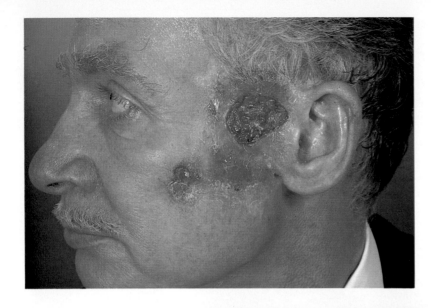

BASAL-CELL CARCINOMA.
Male; *age* 62 years; *duration*
10 years; preauricular area;
confirmed by biopsy.

BASAL-CELL CARCINOMA.
Male; *age* 62 years; *duration*
10 years; preauricular area;
confirmed by biopsy. (Same
patient as in previous photograph.)

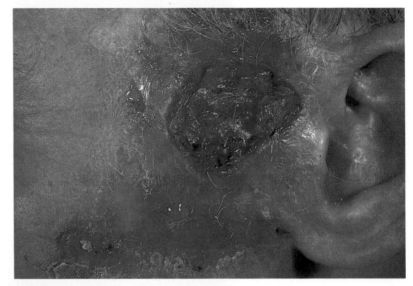

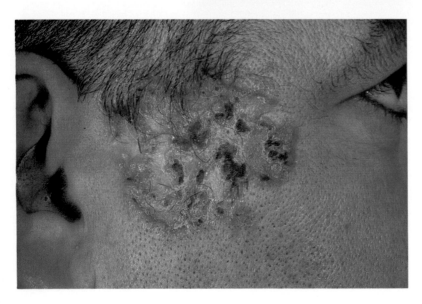

**BASAL-CELL CARCINOMA,
FIELD-FIRE.** Male; *age* 38
years; *duration* 9 years; temple; confirmed by biopsy.

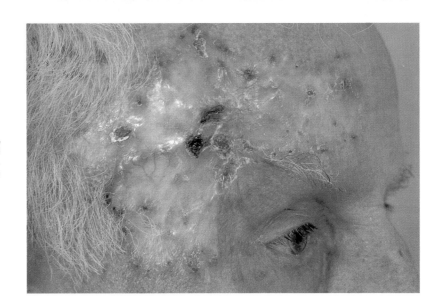

BASAL-CELL CARCINOMA, FIELD-FIRE. Male; *age* 88 years; *duration* 20 years; forehead, temple; confirmed by biopsy.

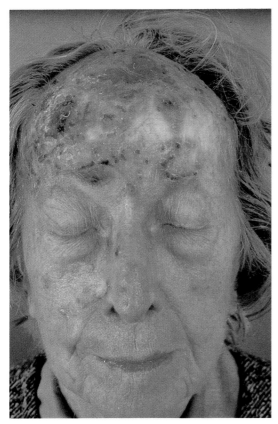

BASAL-CELL CARCINOMA, FIELD-FIRE. Female; *age* 65 years; *duration* 17 years; forehead and frontal area; confirmed by biopsy.

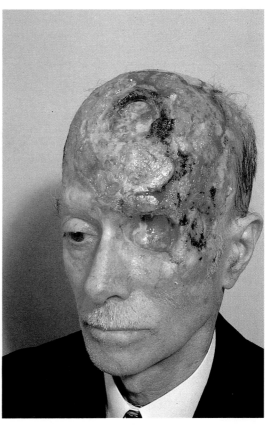

BASAL-CELL CARCINOMA, FIELD-FIRE. Male; *age* 89 years; *duration* many years; scalp, face, orbit; confirmed by biopsy.

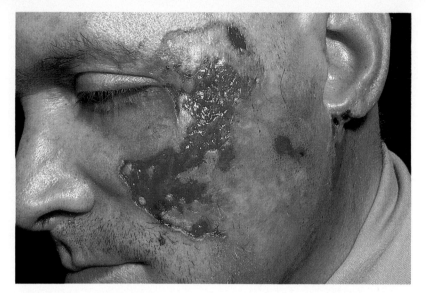

BASAL-CELL CARCINOMA, FIELD-FIRE. Male; *age* 60 years; *duration* 20 years; temple, cheek, ear; confirmed by biopsy.

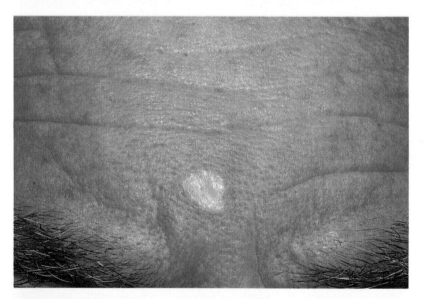

BASAL-CELL CARCINOMA, MORPHEA-LIKE. Male; *age* 65 years; *duration* 10 years; forehead; confirmed by biopsy.

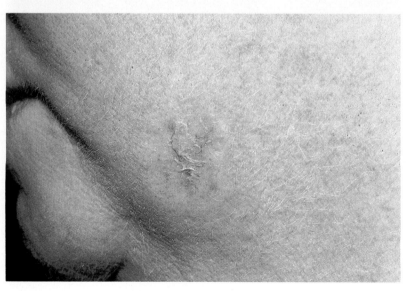

BASAL-CELL CARCINOMA, MORPHEA-LIKE. Female; *age* 50 years; *duration* 3 years; cheek; confirmed by biopsy.

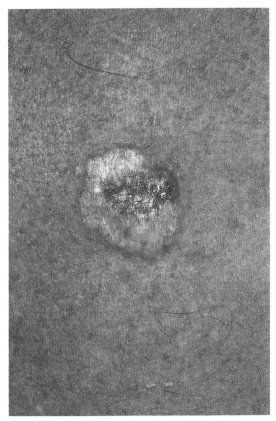

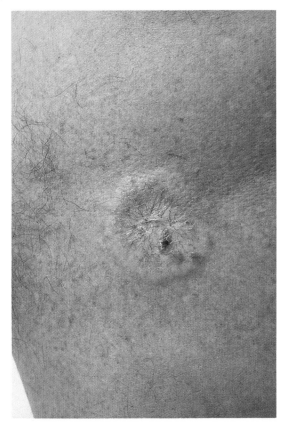

BASAL-CELL CARCINOMA, MORPHEA-LIKE. Male; *age* 51 years; scapular area; confirmed by biopsy.

BASAL-CELL CARCINOMA, MORPHEA-LIKE. *Age* 57 years; scapular area; confirmed by biopsy.

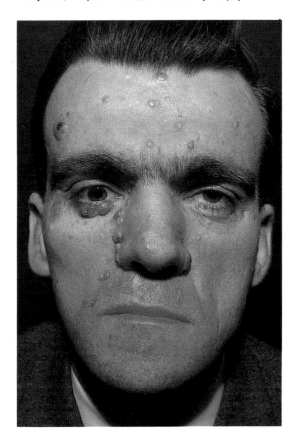

BASAL-CELL CARCINOMAS, NEVOID. Male; *age* 39 years; face; confirmed by biopsy.

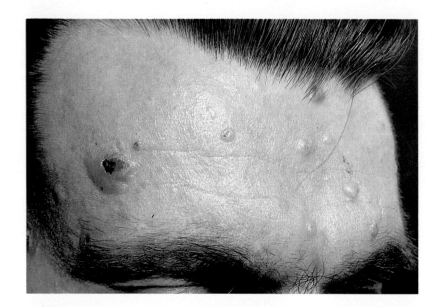

BASAL-CELL CARCINOMAS, NEVOID. Male; *age* 39 years; forehead; confirmed by biopsy.

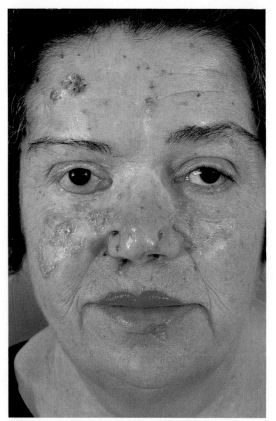

BASAL-CELL CARCINOMAS, NEVOID. Female; *age* 60 years; *duration* 15 years; face; confirmed by biopsy.

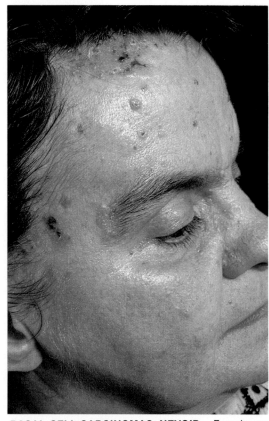

BASAL-CELL CARCINOMAS, NEVOID. Female; *age* 58 years; *duration* 30 years; confirmed by biopsy.

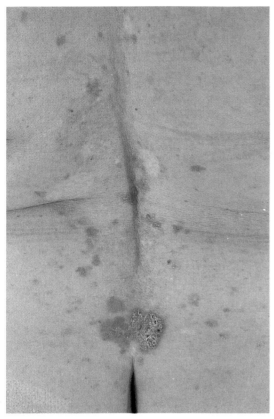

BASAL-CELL CARCINOMAS, NEVOID. Female; *age* 58 years; *duration* 30 years; back; confirmed by biopsy.

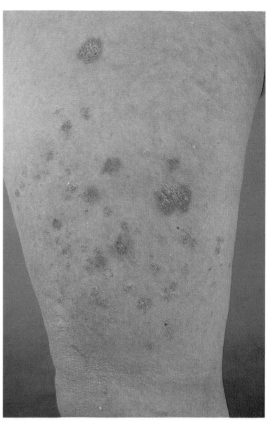

BASAL-CELL CARCINOMAS, NEVOID. Female; *age* 58 years; *duration* 30 years; leg; confirmed by biopsy.

BASAL-CELL CARCINOMA, NEVOID (PINK PALMAR PITS). Female; *age* 58 years; *duration* 30 years.

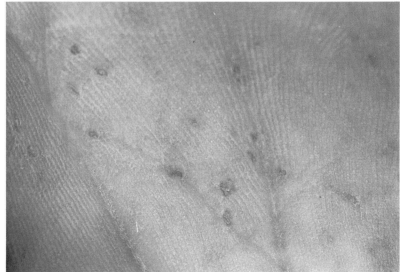

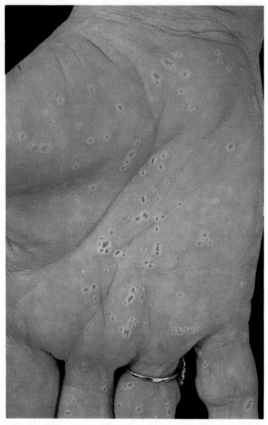

BASAL-CELL CARCINOMA, NEVOID (PINK PALMAR PITS, AFTER SOAKING). Female; *age* 58 years; *duration* 30 years.

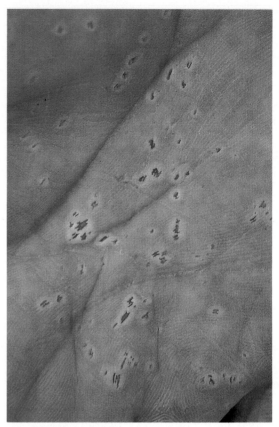

BASAL-CELL CARCINOMA, NEVOID (PINK PALMAR PITS, AFTER SOAKING). Female; *age* 58 years; *duration* 30 years.

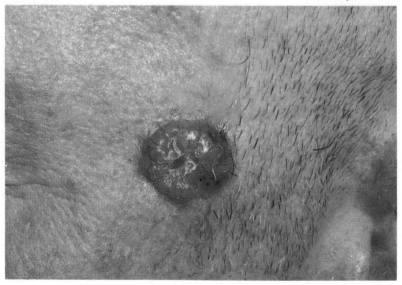

BASAL-CELL CARCINOMA, NODULAR. Male; *age* 61 years; temple; confirmed by biopsy.

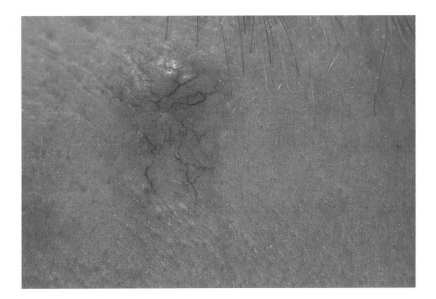

BASAL-CELL CARCINOMA, NODULAR. Female; *age* 58 years; *duration* 3 years; forehead; confirmed by biopsy.

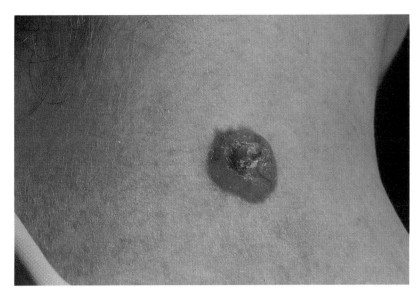

BASAL-CELL CARCINOMA, NODULAR. Female; *age* 36 years; *duration* 2 years; nuchal area; confirmed by biopsy.

BASAL-CELL CARCINOMA, NODULAR. Female; *age* 49 years; *duration* 4 months; nuchal area; confirmed by biopsy.

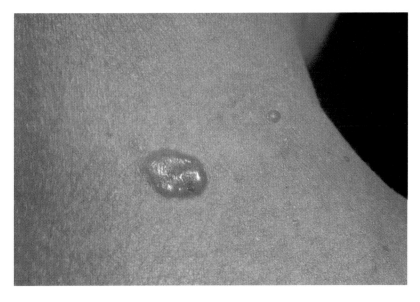

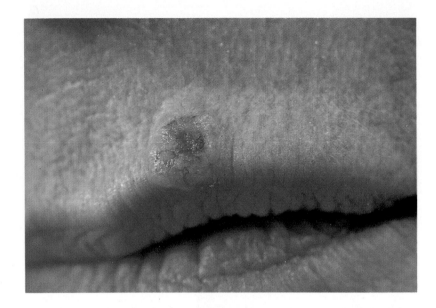

BASAL-CELL CARCINOMA, NODULAR. Female; *age* 55 years; *duration* 12 years; lip; confirmed by biopsy.

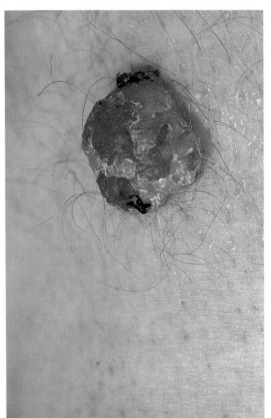

BASAL-CELL CARCINOMA, NODULAR. Male; *age* 67 years; *duration* 11 years; leg; confirmed by biopsy.

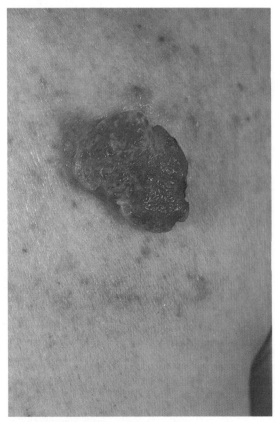

BASAL-CELL CARCINOMA, NODULAR. Male; *age* 49 years; back; confirmed by biopsy.

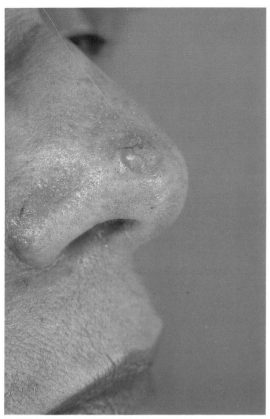

BASAL-CELL CARCINOMA, NODULAR. Female; *age* 56 years; nose; confirmed by biopsy.

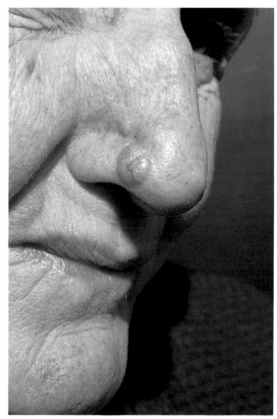

BASAL-CELL CARCINOMA, NODULAR. Female; *age* 68 years; *duration* 14 months; nose; confirmed by biopsy.

BASAL-CELL CARCINOMA, NODULAR. Female; *age* 49 years; *duration* 17 years; nose; confirmed by biopsy.

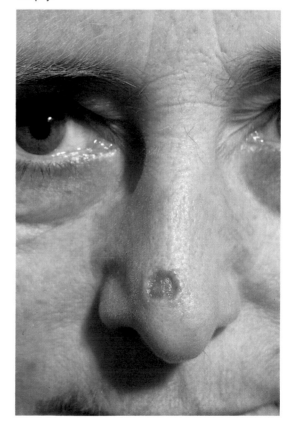

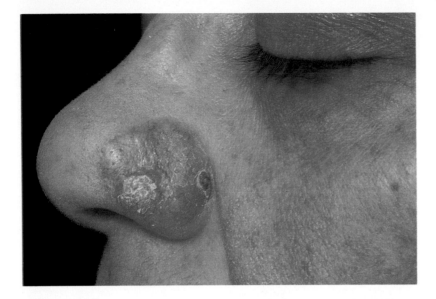

BASAL-CELL CARCINOMA, NODULAR. Female; *age 55* years; *duration* 38 years; ala nasi; confirmed by biopsy.

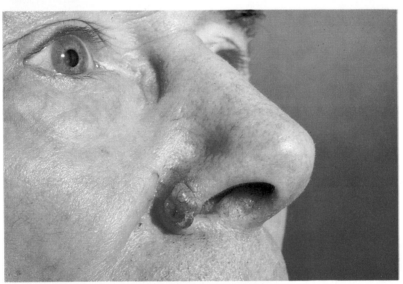

BASAL-CELL CARCINOMA, NODULAR. Male; *age 72* years; *duration* 2 years; ala nasi; confirmed by biopsy.

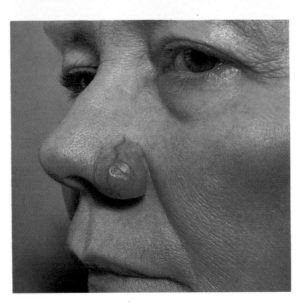

BASAL-CELL CARCINOMA, NODULAR. Female; *age 32* years; *duration* 3 years; ala nasi; confirmed by biopsy.

BASAL-CELL CARCINOMA, NODULAR. Female; nose.

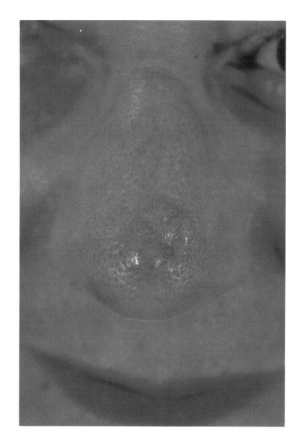

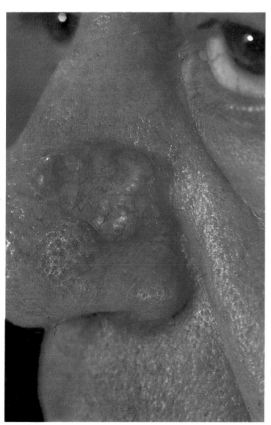

BASAL-CELL CARCINOMA, NODULAR. Male; *age* 65 years; *duration* 7 years; nose; confirmed by biopsy.

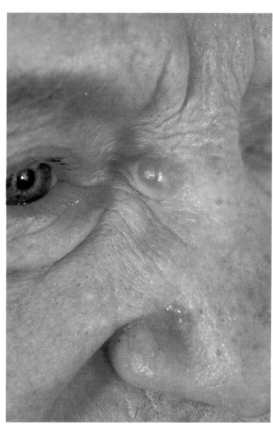

BASAL-CELL CARCINOMAS, NODULAR. Female; *age* 68 years; *duration* 4 months; inner canthus; confirmed by biopsy.

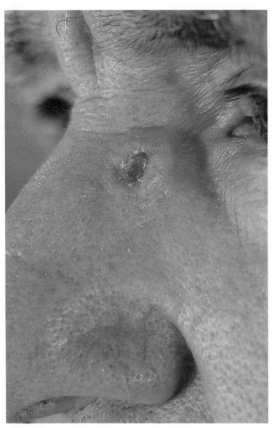

BASAL-CELL CARCINOMA, NODULAR. Male; *age* 70 years; *duration* 2 years; nose; confirmed by biopsy.

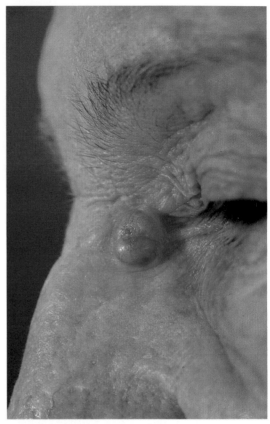

BASAL-CELL CARCINOMA, NODULAR. Female; *age* 50 years; bridge of nose; confirmed by biopsy.

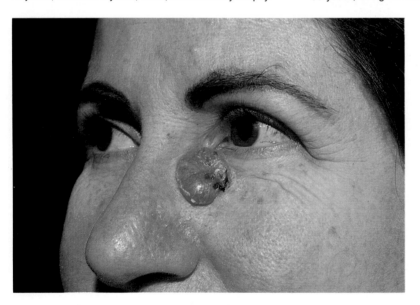

BASAL-CELL CARCINOMA, NODULAR. Female, *age* 45 years; *duration* 7 years; below inner canthus; confirmed by biopsy.

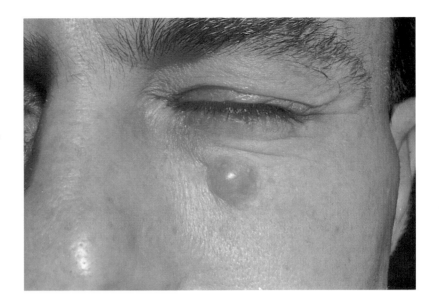

BASAL-CELL CARCINOMA, NODULAR. Male; *age* 33 years; *duration* 13 months; malar area; confirmed by biopsy.

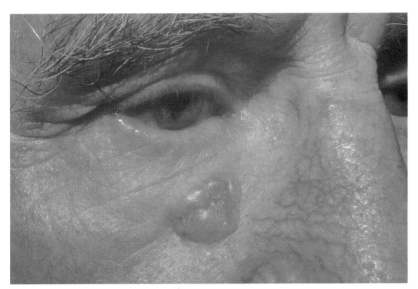

BASAL-CELL CARCINOMA, NODULAR. Male; *age* 75 years; *duration* 4 years; cheek; confirmed by biopsy.

BASAL-CELL CARCINOMA, NODULAR. Male; *age* 64 years; *duration* 3 years; upper and lower eyelids; confirmed by biopsy.

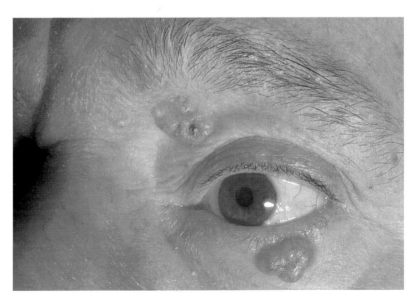

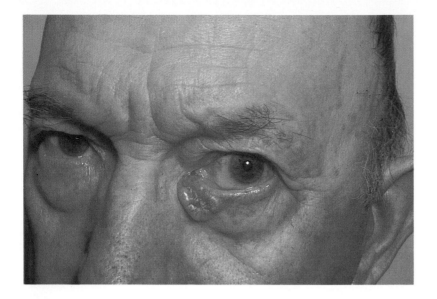

BASAL-CELL CARCINOMA, NODULAR. Male; inner canthus and lower eyelid; conformed by biopsy.

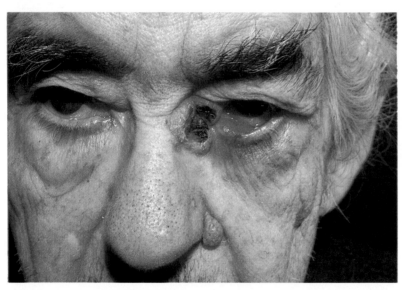

BASAL-CELL CARCINOMA, NODULAR. Male; *age* 84 years; *duration* 5 years; inner canthal area; confirmed by biopsy.

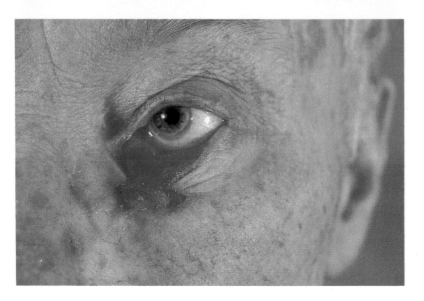

BASAL-CELL CARCINOMA, NODULAR. Male; *age* 71 years; *duration* 10 years; lower eyelid and cheek; confirmed by biopsy.

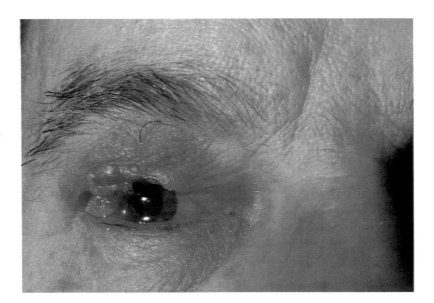

BASAL-CELL CARCINOMA, NODULAR. Male; *age* 58 years; *duration* 4 years; upper and lower eyelid; confirmed by biopsy.

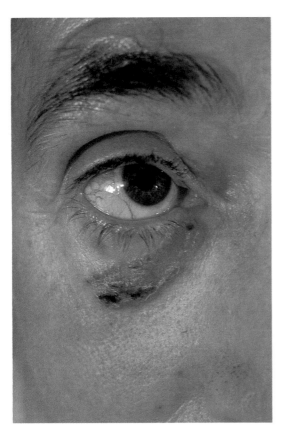

BASAL-CELL CARCINOMA, NODULAR. Male; lower eyelid.

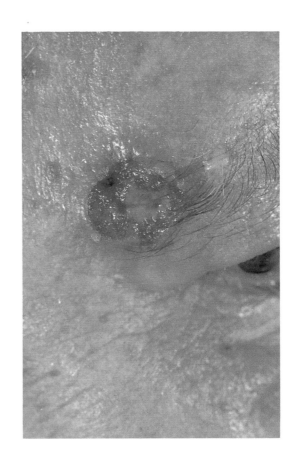

BASAL-CELL CARCINOMA, NODULAR. Female; *age* 70 years; *duration* 13 months; eyebrow; confirmed by biopsy.

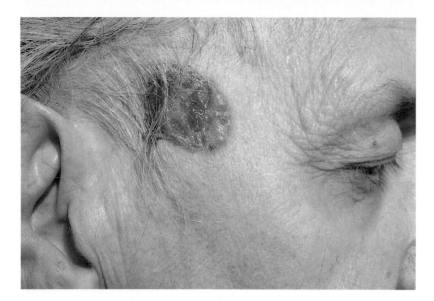

BASAL-CELL CARCINOMA, NODULAR. Female; *age* 78 years; *duration* 3 years; temple; confirmed by biopsy.

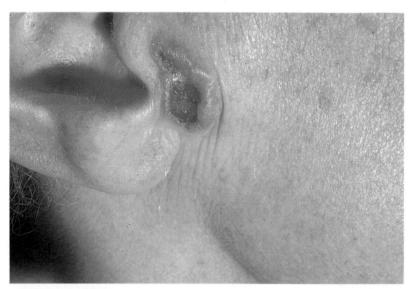

BASAL-CELL CARCINOMA, NODULAR. Female; *age* 71 years; *duration* 3 years; preauricular area.

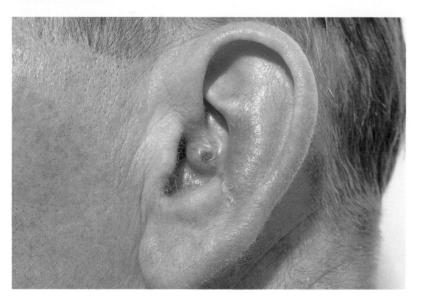

BASAL-CELL CARCINOMA, NODULAR. Male; *age* 44 years; concha of ear; confirmed by biopsy.

BASAL-CELL CARCINOMA, NODULAR. Male; *age* 74 years; *duration* 13 months; ear; confirmed by biopsy.

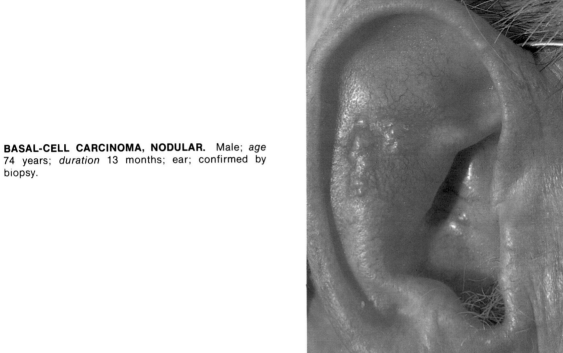

BASAL-CELL CARCINOMA, NODULAR. Female; *age* 71 years; *duration* 4 months; ear; confirmed by biopsy.

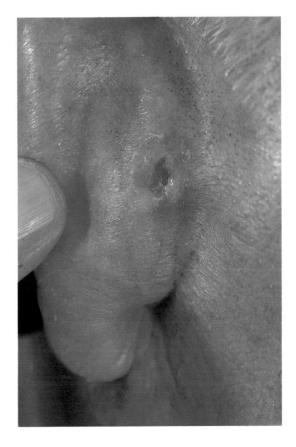

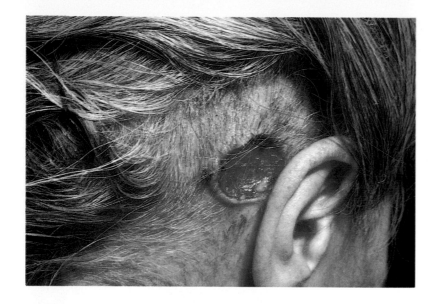

BASAL-CELL CARCINOMA, NODULAR. Female; *age* 60 years; *duration* 3 years; retro-auricular area; confirmed by biopsy.

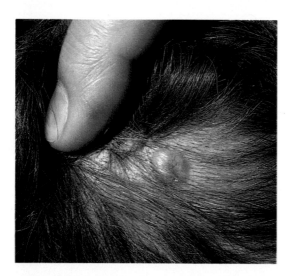

BASAL-CELL CARCINOMA, NODULAR. Male; *age* 55 years; *duration* 7 months; scalp; confirmed by biopsy.

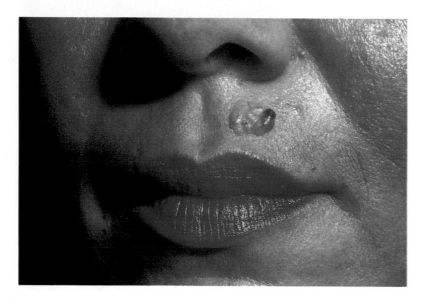

BASAL-CELL CARCINOMA, NODULAR. Female, *age* 36 years; upper lip; confirmed by biopsy.

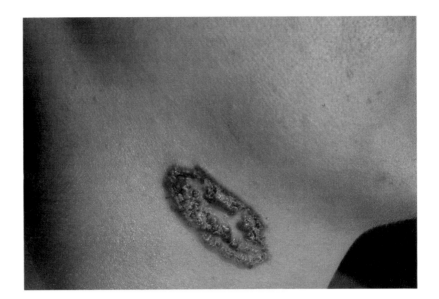

BASAL-CELL CARCINOMA, PIGMENTED. Female; *age* 32 years; *duration* 3 years; neck; confirmed by biopsy.

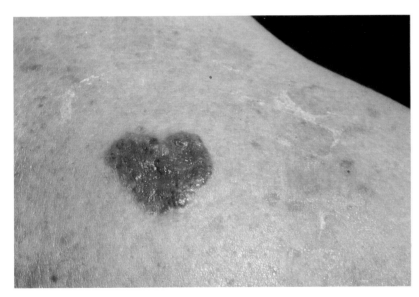

BASAL-CELL CARCINOMA, PIGMENTED. Male; *age* 63 years; *duration* 2 years; suprascapular; confirmed by biopsy.

BASAL-CELL CARCINOMA, PIGMENTED. Male; *age* 61 years; *duration* 2 years; confirmed by biopsy.

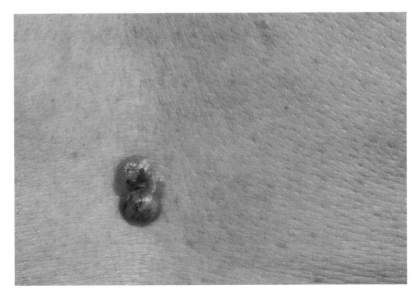

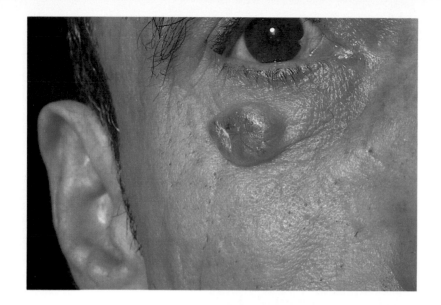

BASAL-CELL CARCINOMA, PIGMENTED. Male; *age* 61 years; *duration* 13 months; eyelid; confirmed by biopsy.

BASAL-CELL CARCINOMA, PIGMENTED. Male; *age* 53 years; *duration* 8 years; cheek; confirmed by biopsy.

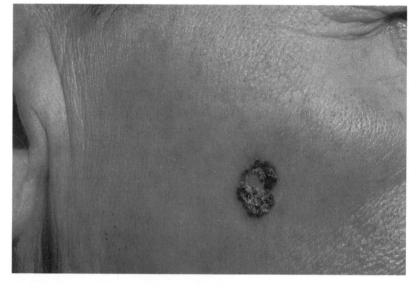

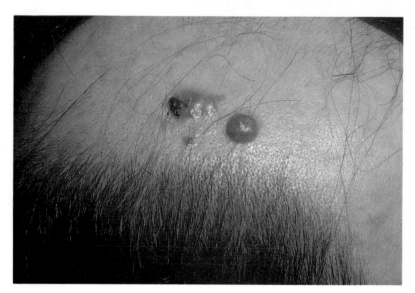

BASAL-CELL CARCINOMA, PIGMENTED. Male; *age* 38 years; scalp; confirmed by biopsy.

BASAL-CELL, PIGMENTED.
Female; *age* 72 years; *duration* 3 years; chin; confirmed by biopsy.

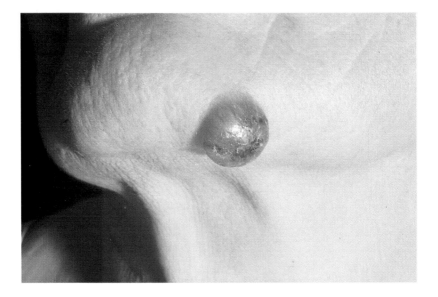

BASAL-CELL CARCINOMA, SUPERFICIAL. Female; *age* 59 years; *duration* more than 20 years; lower back; confirmed by biopsy.

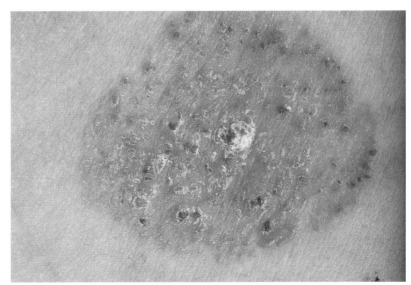

BASAL-CELL CARCINOMA, SUPERFICIAL. Male; *age* 55 years; *duration* 4 years; abdomen; confirmed by biopsy.

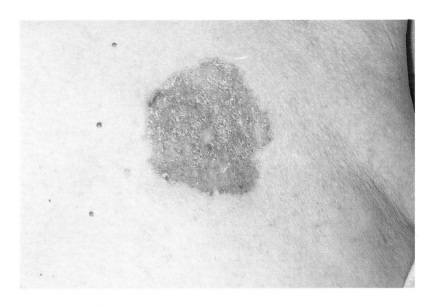

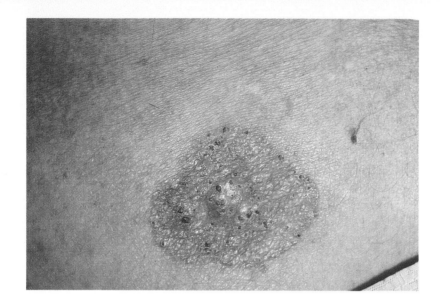

BASAL-CELL CARCINOMA, SUPERFICIAL. Male; *age* 60 years; *duration* 3 years; back; confirmed by biopsy.

BASAL-CELL CARCINOMA, SUPERFICIAL. Male, *age* 77 years; *duration* 10 years; sacral area; confirmed by biopsy.

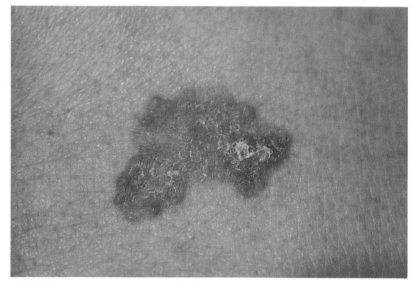

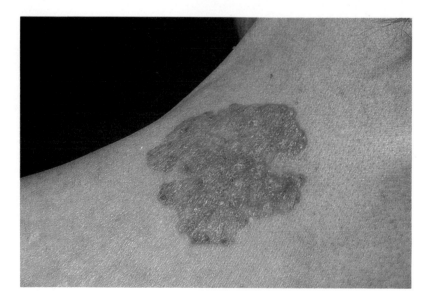

BASAL-CELL CARCINOMA, SUPERFICIAL. Female, *age* 53 years; *duration* 10 years; shoulder; confirmed by biopsy.

BASAL-CELL CARCINOMA, SUPERFICIAL. Male; *age* 63 years; *duration* 7 years; arm; confirmed by biopsy.

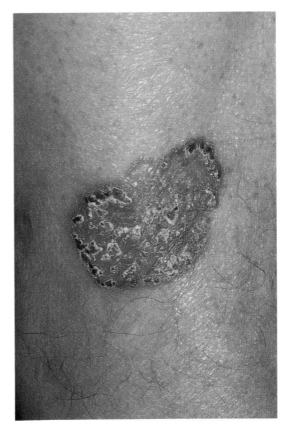

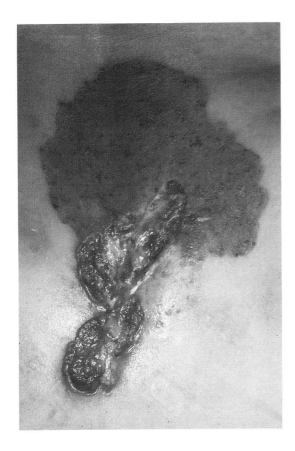

BASAL-CELL CARCINOMA, SUPERFICIAL AND NODULAR. Female; *age* 68 years; *duration* 5 years; sacral area; confirmed by biopsy.

BASAL-CELL CARCINOMA, SUPERFICIAL AND NODULAR. Male; *age* 65 years; *duration* 13 years; lower back; confirmed by biopsy.

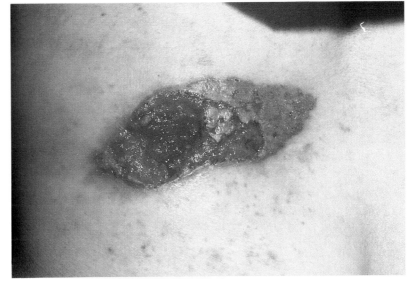

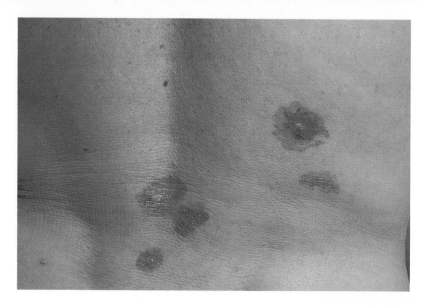

BASAL-CELL CARCINOMAS, SUPERFICIAL. Male; *age* 60 years; *duration* 3 years; back; confirmed by biopsy.

BASAL-CELL CARCINOMAS, SUPERFICIAL. Female; *age* 58 years; *duration* 15 years; back; confirmed by biopsy.

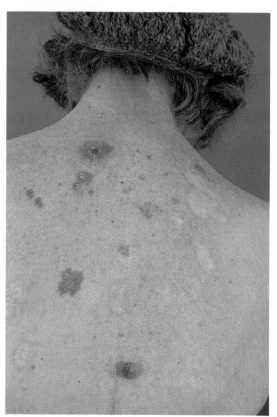

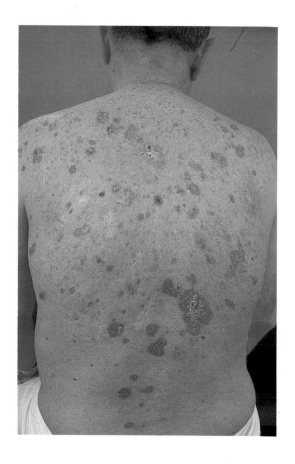

BASAL-CELL CARCINOMA, SUPERFICIAL. Male; *age* 65 years; back; confirmed by biopsy.

BASAL-SQUAMOUS CELL CARCINOMA. Female; *age* 77 years; *duration* 6 years; chin; confirmed by biopsy.

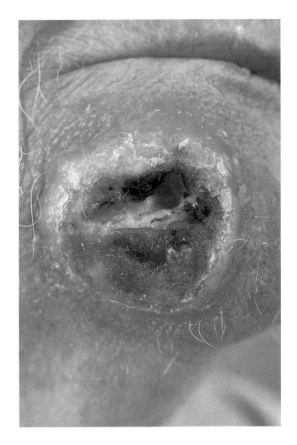

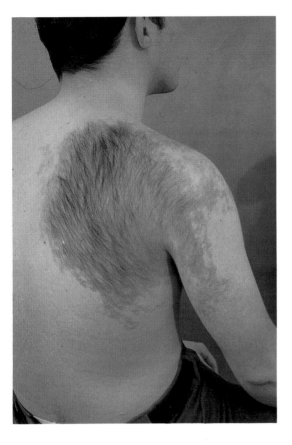

BECKER'S NEVUS. Male; *age* 17 years; *duration* 11 years; trunk and arm.

BECKER'S NEVUS. Male; *age* 16 years; *duration* 3 years; suprascapular area.

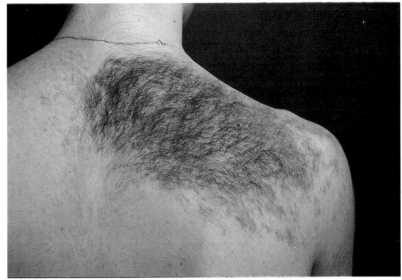

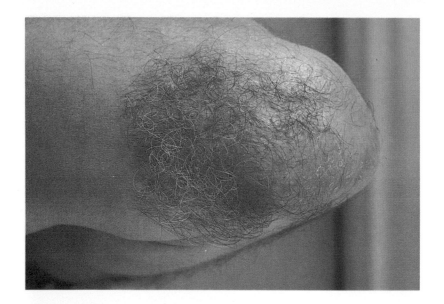

BECKER'S NEVUS. Male; *age* 55 years; elbow.

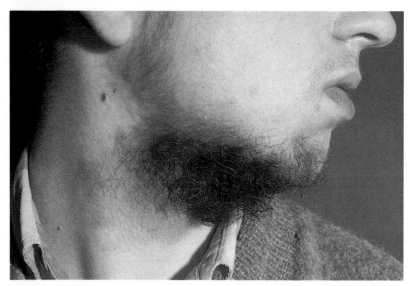

BECKER'S NEVUS. Male; *age* 14 years; *duration* 13 years; right submandibular area and neck; confirmed by biopsy.

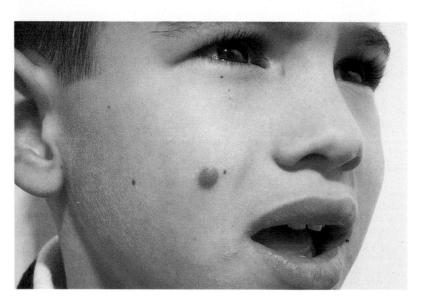

BENIGN JUVENILE MELA-NOMA. Cheek; confirmed by biopsy.

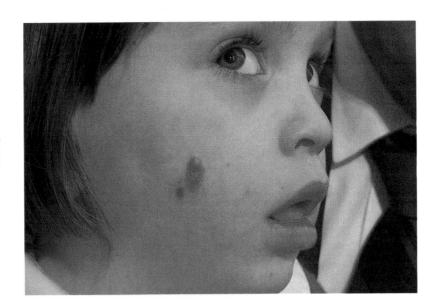

BENIGN JUVENILE MELA-NOMA. Female; *age* 3 years; *duration* 6 months; cheek; confirmed by biopsy.

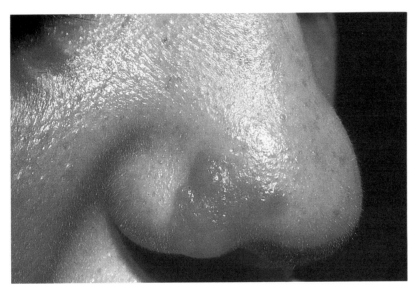

BENIGN JUVENILE MELA-NOMA. Female; nose; confirmed by biopsy.

BENIGN JUVENILE MELA-NOMA. Female; adult; confirmed by biopsy.

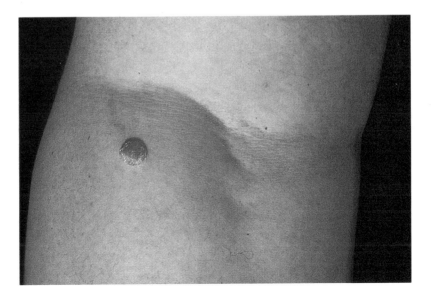

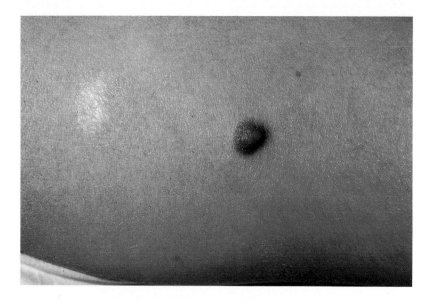

**BENIGN JUVENILE MELA-
NOMA.** Male; arm; confirmed
by biopsy.

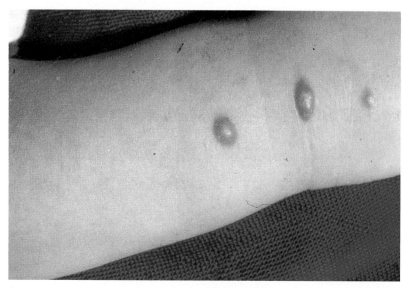

**BENIGN JUVENILE MELA-
NOMA (MULTIPLE AND AG-
MINATED).** Female; wrist;
confirmed by biopsy.

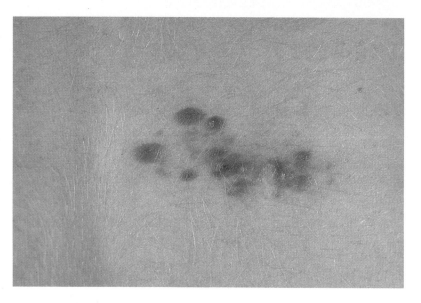

**BENIGN JUVENILE MELA-
NOMA (MULTIPLE AND AG-
MINATED).** Male; *age* 5
years; *duration* since birth;
mid-back; confirmed by biopsy.

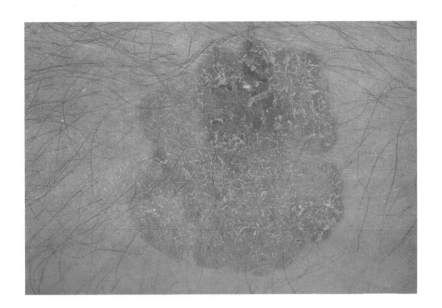

BOWEN'S DISEASE. Male; *age* 46 years; *duration* 8–10 years; chest; confirmed by biopsy.

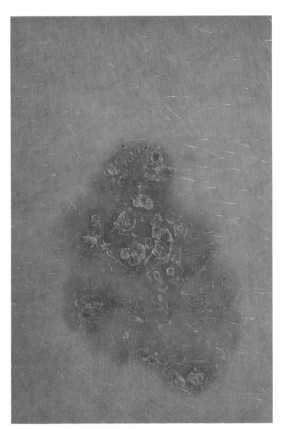

BOWEN'S DISEASE. Female; *age* 54 years; back; confirmed by biopsy.

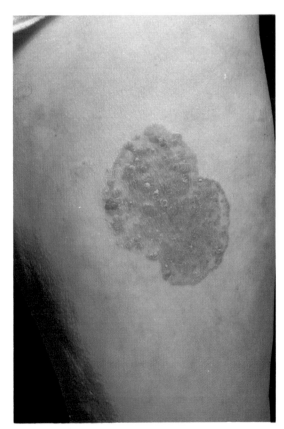

BOWEN'S DISEASE. Male; *age* 76 years; *duration* 12 years; confirmed by biopsy.

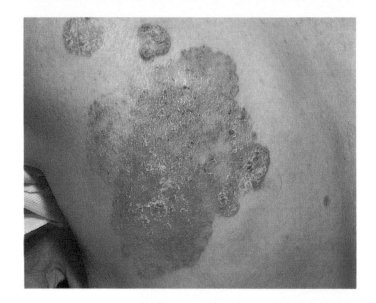

BOWEN'S DISEASE. Male; back; confirmed by biopsy.

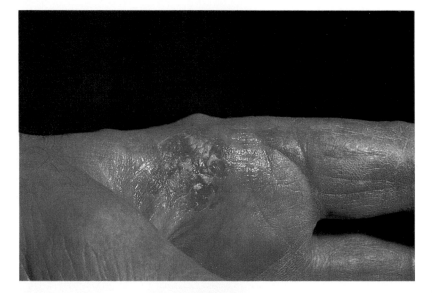

BOWEN'S DISEASE. Male; *age* 63 years; *duration* 2 years; hand; confirmed by biopsy.

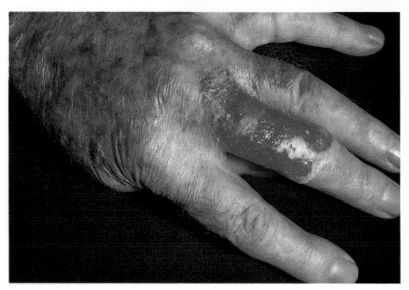

BOWEN'S DISEASE. Male; *age* 83 years; *duration* 5 years; finger; confirmed by biopsy.

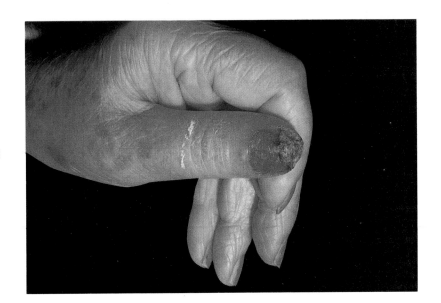

BOWEN'S DISEASE. Female; nailbed of thumb.

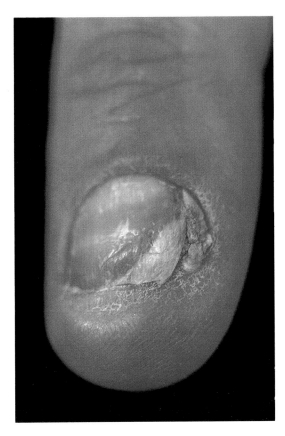

BOWEN'S DISEASE. Nailbed.

BOWEN'S DISEASE. Male; *age* 50 years; peri- and sub-ungual areas; confirmed by biopsy.

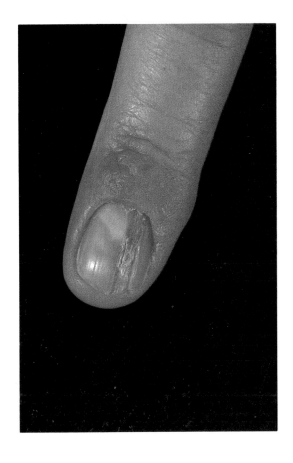

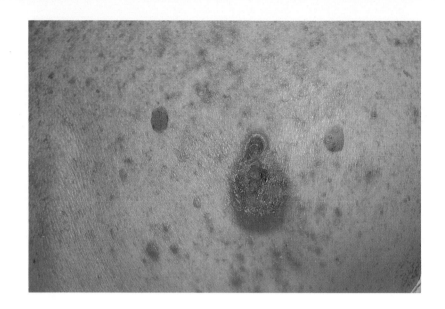

BOWEN'S DISEASE. Female; *age* 69 years; *duration* 4 months; scapular area; confirmed by biopsy.

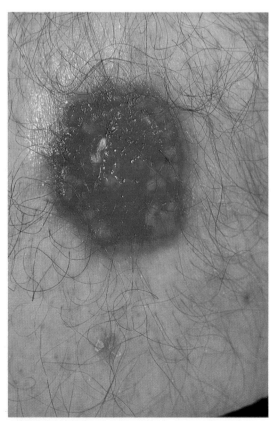

BOWEN'S DISEASE, INVASIVE. Male; *age* 46 years; *duration* 8 years; leg; confirmed by biopsy.

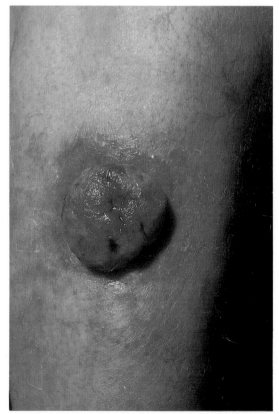

BOWEN'S DISEASE, INVASIVE. Male; *age* 54 years; *duration* 18 months; leg; confirmed by biopsy.

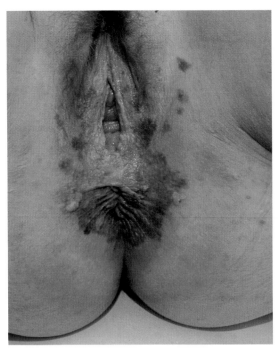

BOWEN'S DISEASE. Female; *age* 30 years; *duration* 2 years; anogenital area.

BOWEN'S DISEASE. Female; *age* 49 years; *duration* 10 years; anogenital area; confirmed by biopsy.

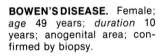

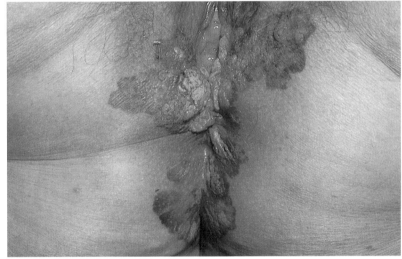

BRANCHIAL CLEFT SINUS. Female; *age* 5 years; *duration* since birth; mandibular area.

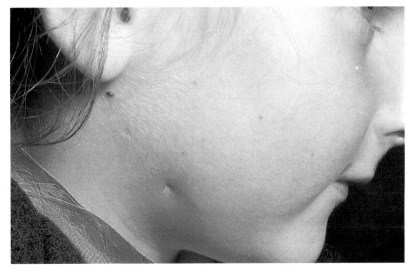

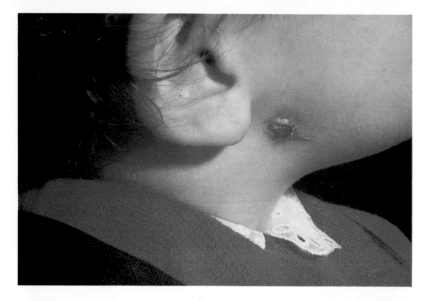

BRANCHIAL CLEFT SINUS.
Female; *duration* since birth;
mandibular area.

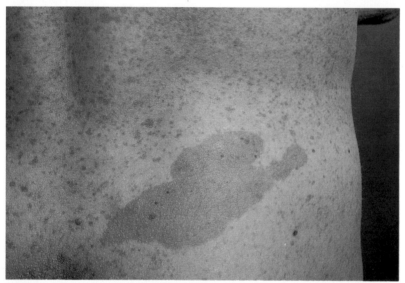

CAFE-AU-LAIT SPOT. Male;
age 17 years; *duration* since
birth; buttock; confirmed by
biopsy.

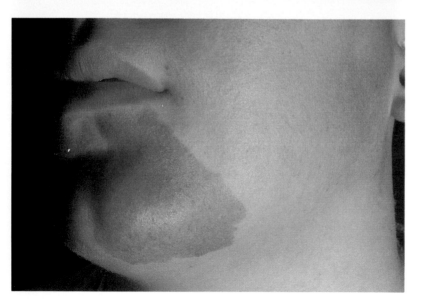

CAFE-AU-LAIT SPOT. Male;
age 11 years; chin; confirmed
by biopsy.

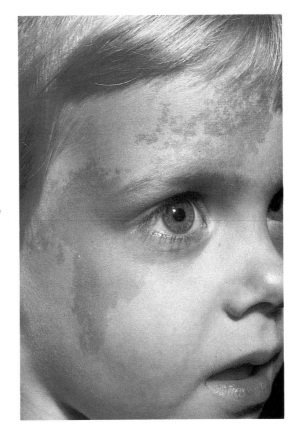

CAFE-AU-LAIT SPOT. Female; *age* 5 years; *duration* since birth; face; confirmed by biopsy.

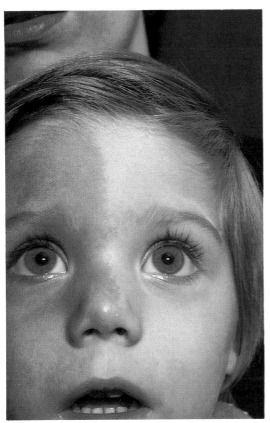

CAFE-AU-LAIT SPOT. Female; *age* 3 years; *duration* 28 months; face.

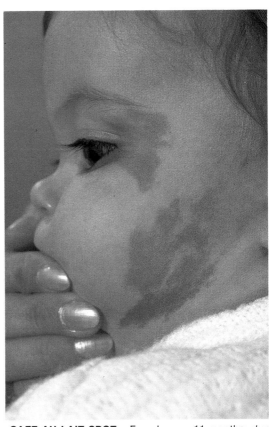

CAFE-AU-LAIT-SPOT. Female; *age* 11 months; *duration* since birth; face.

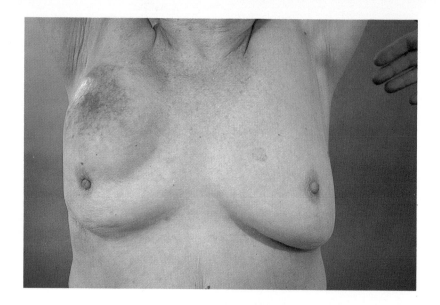

CARCINOMA OF BREAST.
Female.

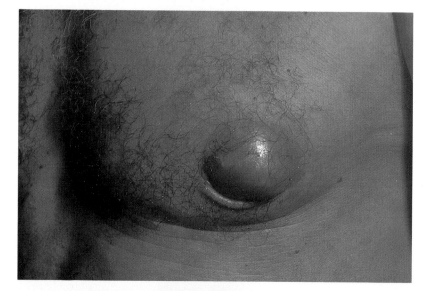

CARCINOMA OF BREAST.
Male; *age* 83 years; *duration* 5
years; breast; confirmed by
biopsy.

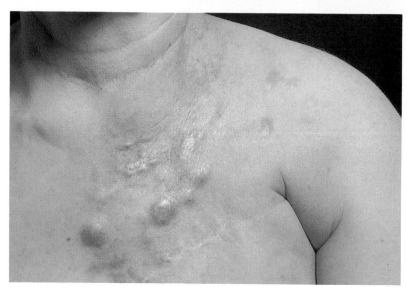

**CARCINOMA OF BREAST,
METASTATIC TO SKIN.** Female; *age* 63 years; *duration*
7 months; chest; confirmed by
biopsy.

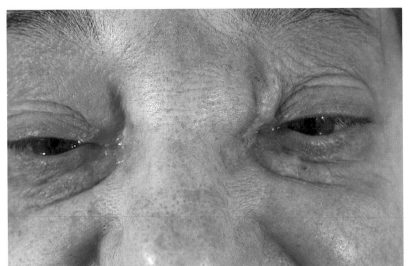

CARCINOMA OF PARA-NASAL SINUS. Female; *age* 67 years; *duration* 1 year; bridge of nose; confirmed by biopsy.

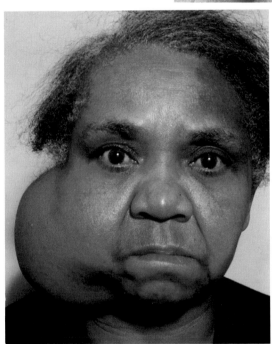

CARCINOMA OF PAROTID GLAND. Female; *age* 66 years; *duration* 25 years; neck.

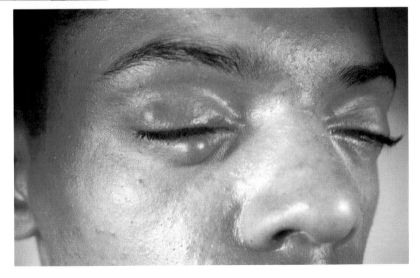

CHALAZIONS. Male; eyelids.

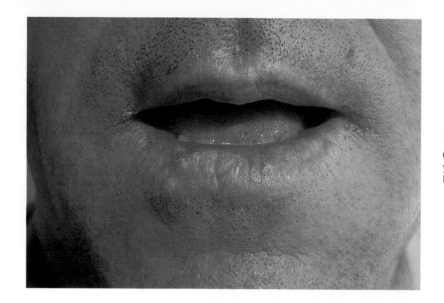

CHEILITIS GLANDULARIS WITH SQUAMOUS-CELL CARCINOMA. Male; *age* 46 years; lower lip; confirmed by biopsy.

CHEILITIS GLANDULARIS WITH SQUAMOUS-CELL CARCINOMA. Male; *age* 61 years; *duration* 13 months; lower lip; confirmed by biopsy.

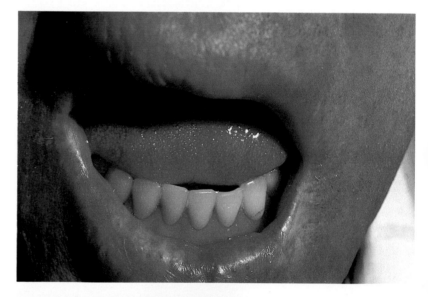

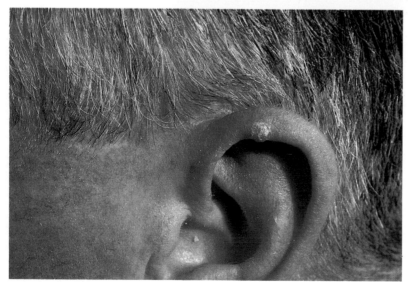

CHONDRODERMATITIS NODULARIS CHRONICA HELICIS. Male; *age* 53 years; *duration* 6 years; helix; confirmed by biopsy.

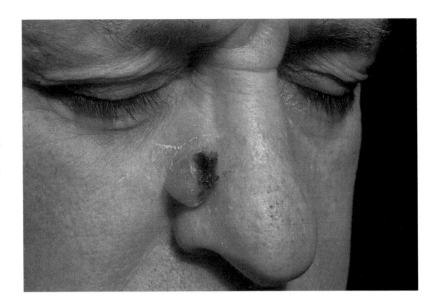

CHONDROID SYRINGOMA (MIXED TUMOR OF SWEAT GLAND). Male; *age* 66 years; *duration* 3 years; nose; confirmed by biopsy.

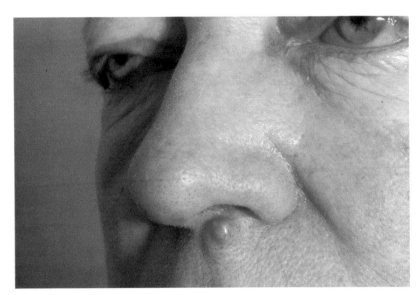

CHONDROID SYRINGOMA (MIXED TUMOR OF SWEAT GLAND). Female; *age* 57 years; *duration* 3 years; upper lip; confirmed by biopsy.

CONNECTIVE TISSUE NEVUS. Male; *age* 5 years; *duration* since birth; abdomen; confirmed by biopsy.

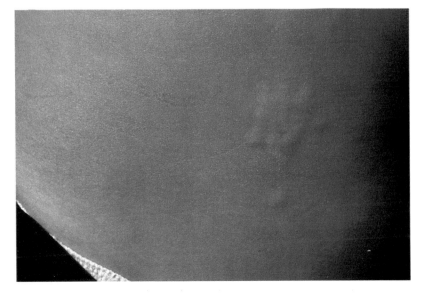

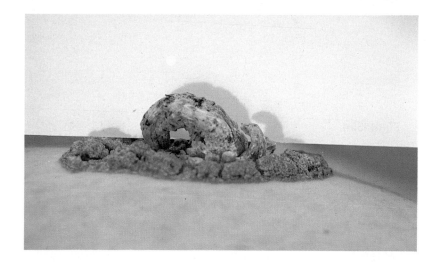

CUTANEOUS HORN, ARISING FROM SEBORRHEIC KERATOSIS. Male; age 64 years; duration 30 years; back; confirmed by biopsy.

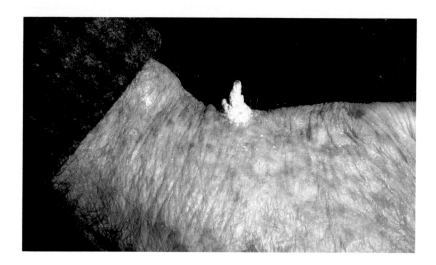

CUTANEOUS HORN, ARISING FROM ACTINIC KERATOSIS. Male; hand; confirmed by biopsy.

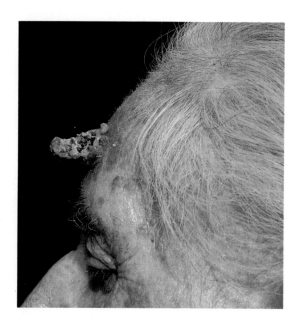

CUTANEOUS HORN, ARISING FROM SQUAMOUS-CELL CARCINOMA. Female; age 68 years; forehead; confirmed by biopsy.

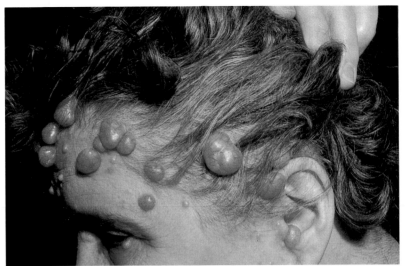

CYLINDROMAS. Female; *age* 58 years; *duration* 18 years; face and scalp; confirmed by biopsy.

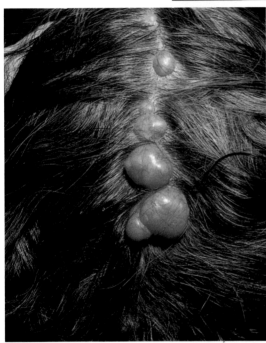

CYLINDROMAS. Female; *age* 58 years; *duration* 18 years; scalp; confirmed by biopsy. (Same patient as in previous photograph.)

CYLINDROMA. Male; *age* 62 years; *duration* 22 years; forehead, scalp; preauricular; confirmed by biopsy.

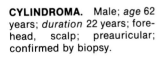

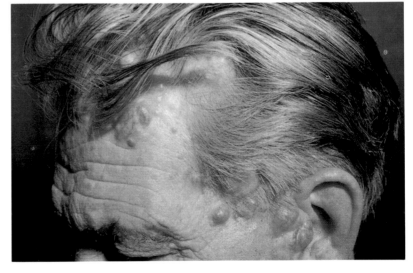

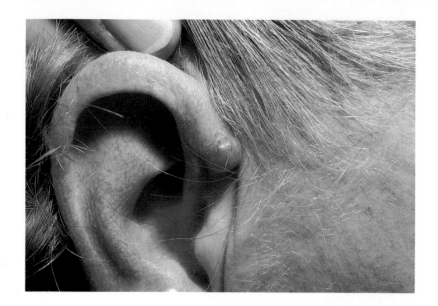

CYLINDROMA. Male; *age* 60 years; *duration* 3 years; ear; confirmed by biopsy.

CYLINDROMA. Female; *age* 61 years; *duration* 5 years; forehead; confirmed by biopsy.

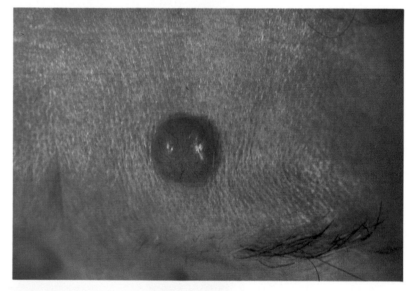

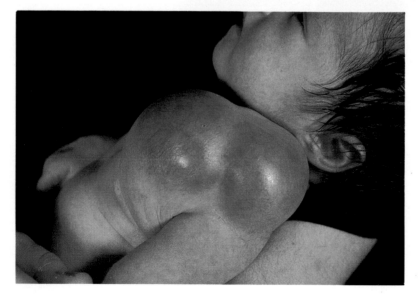

CYSTIC HYGROMA. Shoulder.

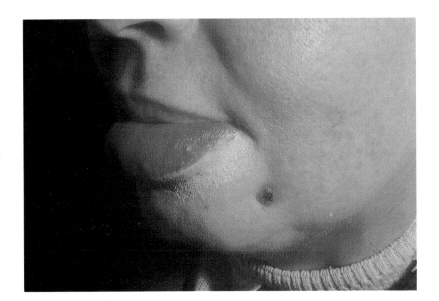

DENTAL SINUS. Female; *age* 38 years; *duration* 6 months; chin; confirmed by biopsy.

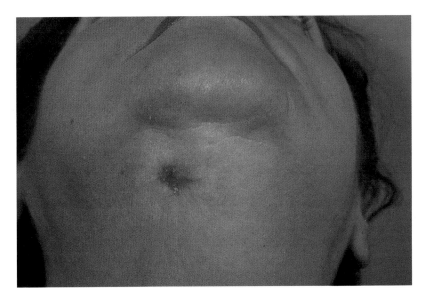

DENTAL SINUS. Female; *age* 57 years; *duration* 1 year; submental area.

DENTAL SINUS. Male; *age* 27 years; *duration* 10 months; chin; confirmed by biopsy.

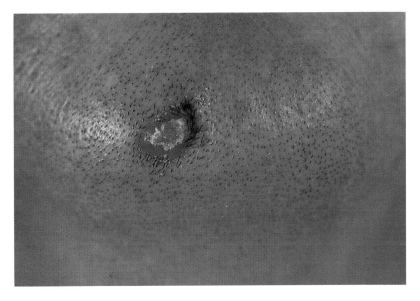

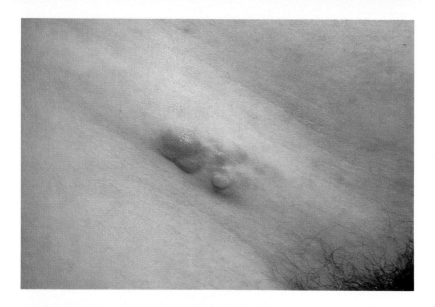

DERMATOFIBROSARCOMA PROTUBERANS. Male; *age* 44 years; *duration* 10 years; confirmed by biopsy.

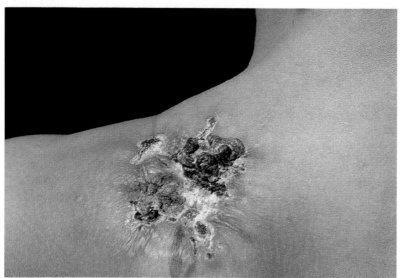

DERMATOFIBROSARCOMA PROTUBERANS. Female; *age* 25 years; *duration* 4 years; shoulder; confirmed by biopsy.

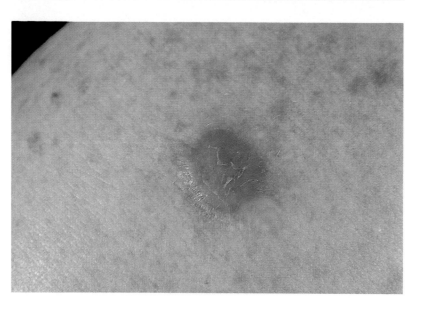

DERMATOFIBROSARCOMA PROTUBERANS. Male; *age* 27 years; shoulder; confirmed by biopsy.

**DERMATOFIBROSARCOMA
PROTUBERANS.** Female;
age 38 years; *duration* 2 years;
deltoid area; confirmed by
biopsy.

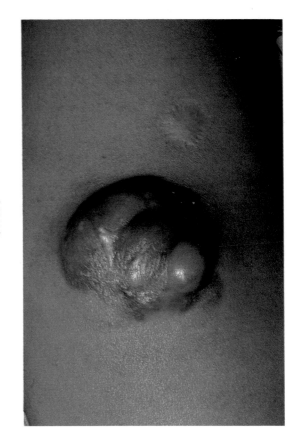

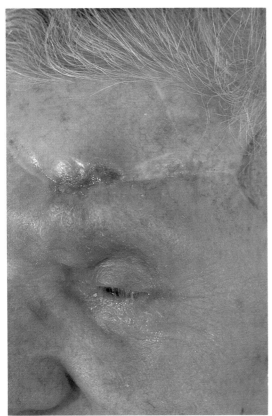

DERMATOFIBROSARCOMA PROTUBERANS. Male;
age 75 years; *duration* 18 months; forehead; confirmed by biopsy.

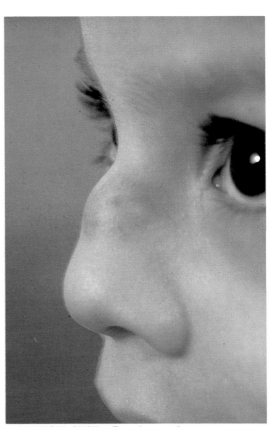

DERMOID CYST. Female; *age* 3 years; nose.

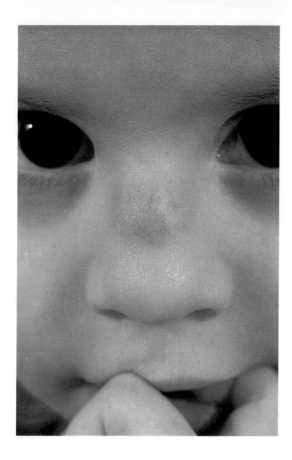

DERMOID CYST. Female; *age* 3 years; bridge of nose. (Same patient as in previous photograph.)

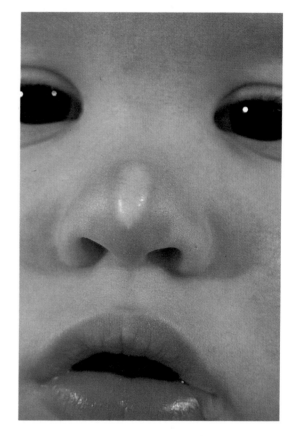

DERMOID CYST. Male; *age* 16 months; nose; confirmed by biopsy.

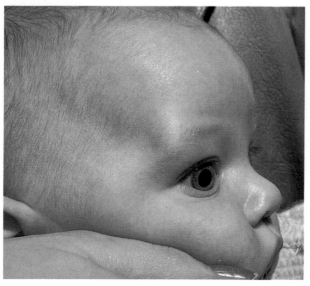

DERMOID CYST. Male; *age* 2 months; *duration* since birth; eyebrow.

DERMOID CYST. Female; *age* 12 years; *duration* 3 months; eyebrow.

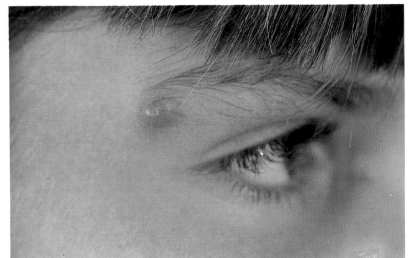

DERMOID CYST. Female; *age* 2 years; *duration* 18 months; upper eyelid; confirmed by biopsy.

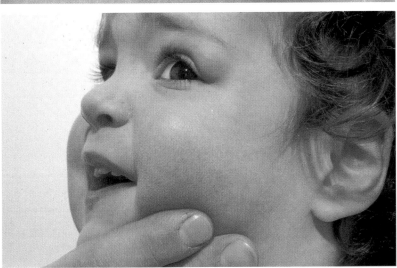

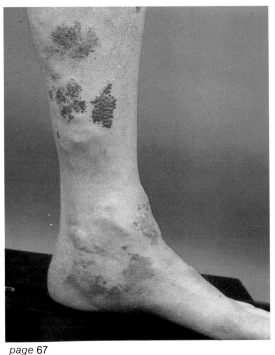

DYSPLASTIC ANGIOPATHY. Male; *age* 41 years; *duration* 5 years; leg; confirmed by biopsy.

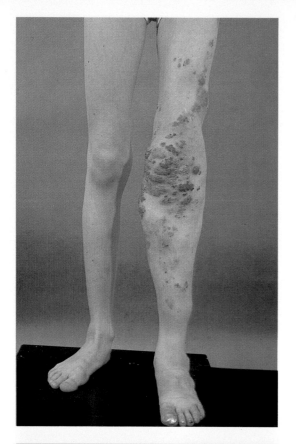

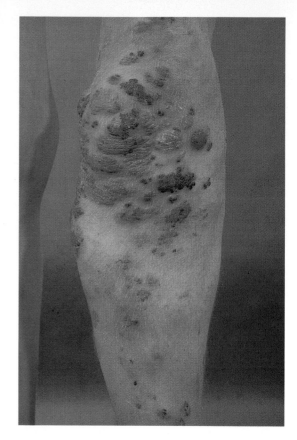

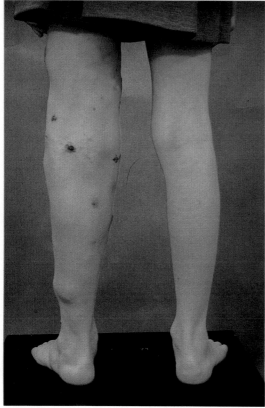

DYSPLASTIC ANGIOPATHY. Female; *age* 9 years; *duration* since birth; lower extremity (*top left*).

DYSPLASTIC ANGIOPATHY. Female; *age* 9 years; *duration* since birth; lower extremity. (Same patient as in previous photograph.) (*top right*).

DYSPLASTIC ANGIOPATHY. Female; *age* 6 years; *duration* since birth; lower extremity.

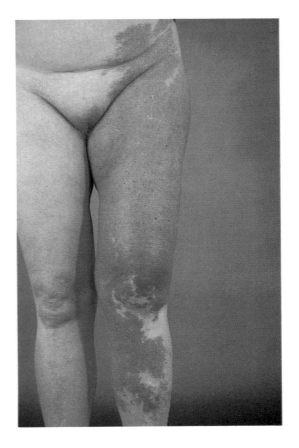

DYSPLASTIC ANGIOPATHY.
Female; *age* 52 years; *duration* since birth; trunk, thigh
and leg.

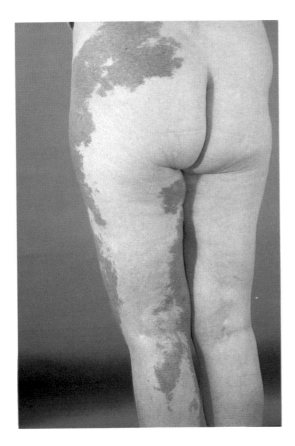

DYSPLASTIC ANGIOPATHY.
Female; *age* 52 years; *duration* since birth; trunk, thigh
and leg. (Same patient as in
previous photograph.)

ECCRINE POROMA. Female;
age 56 years; *duration* 15
years; arch of foot; confirmed
by biopsy.

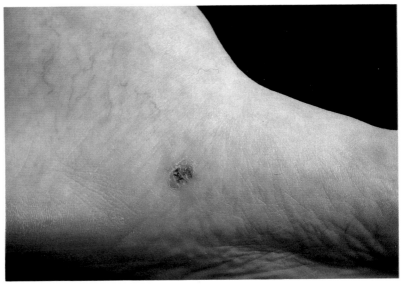

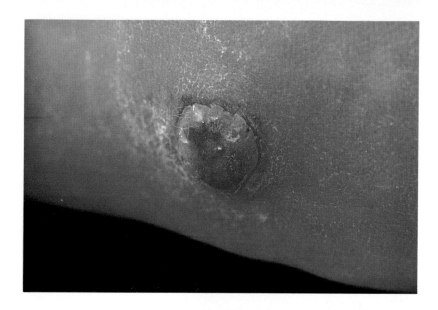

ECCRINE POROMA. Female; *age* 41 years; *duration* 8 years; heel; confirmed by biopsy.

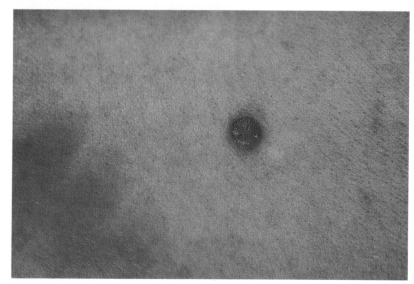

ECCRINE POROMA. Female; *age* 46 years; *duration* 13 months; neck; confirmed by biopsy.

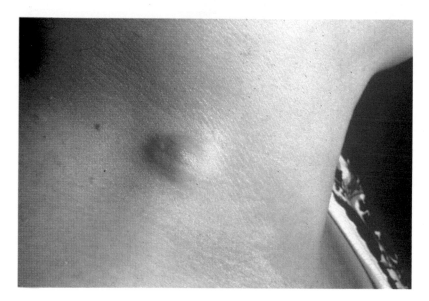

ECCRINE SPIRADENOMA. Female; *age* 42 years; *duration* 5 years; neck; confirmed by biopsy.

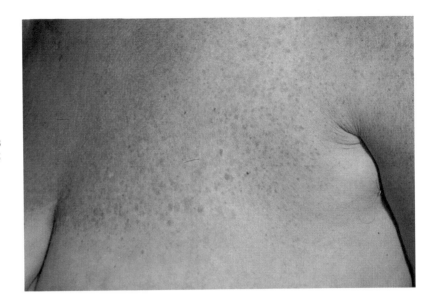

EPHELIDES. Female; *age* 68 years; *duration* "many years"; chest; confirmed by biopsy.

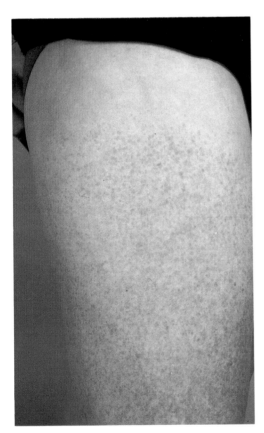

EPHELIDES. Female; *age* 39 years; *duration* years; thigh; confirmed by biopsy.

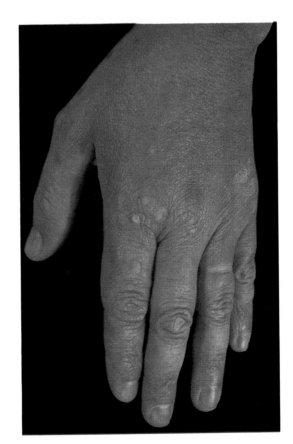

EPIDERMODYSPLASIA VER-RUCIFORMIS. Male; *age* 41 years; *duration* 20 years; hand; confirmed by biopsy.

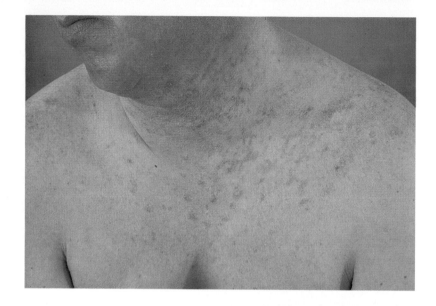

EPIDERMODYSPLASIA VER-RUCIFORMIS. Male; *age* 41 years; *duration* 20 years; neck and chest; confirmed by biopsy.

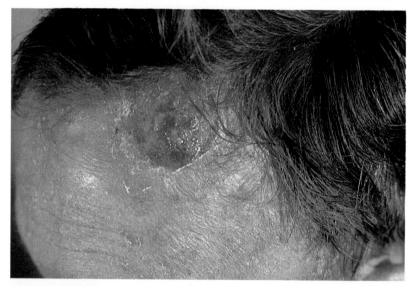

EPIDERMODYSPLASIA VER-RUCIFORMIS WITH SQUA-MOUS-CELL CARCINOMA. Male; *age* 41 years; *duration* 20 years; forehead; confirmed by biopsy. (Same patient as in previous photograph.)

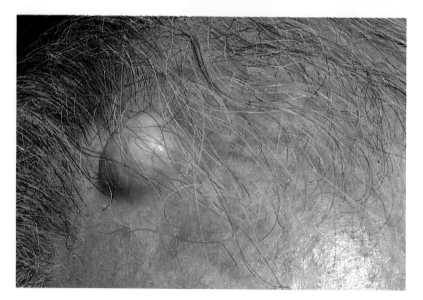

EPITHELIAL CYST. Male; *age* 72 years; *duration* 10 years; temple.

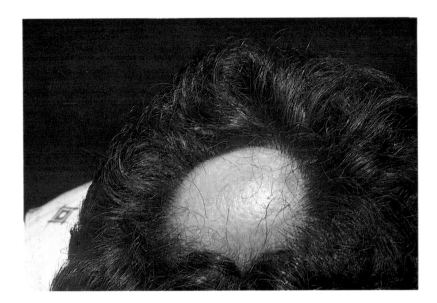

EPITHELIAL CYST. Male; *age* 26 years; scalp; confirmed by biopsy.

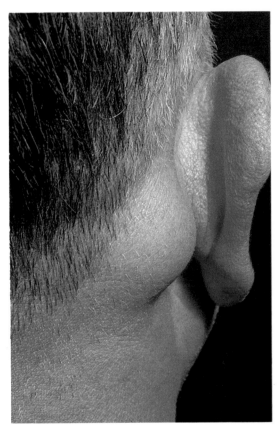

EPITHELIAL CYST. Male; *age* 53 years; *duration* 2 years; postauricular area.

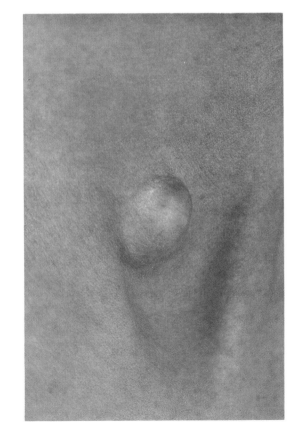

EPITHELIAL CYST. Female; *age* 42 years; *duration* 10 years; neck; confirmed by biopsy.

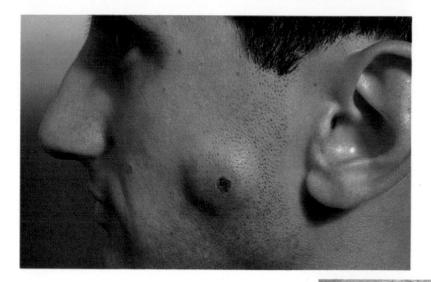

EPITHELIAL CYST. Male; *age* 28 years; *duration* 4 months; cheek.

EPITHELIAL CYSTS. Male; *age* 62 years; scrotum; confirmed by biopsy.

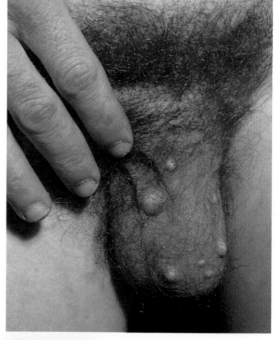

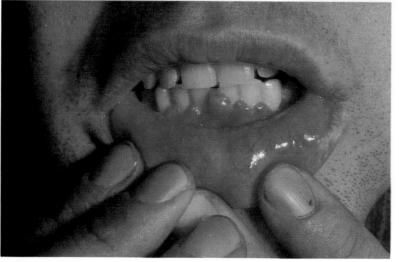

EPULIS. Male; *age* 29 years; *duration* 7 months; gingiva; confirmed by biopsy.

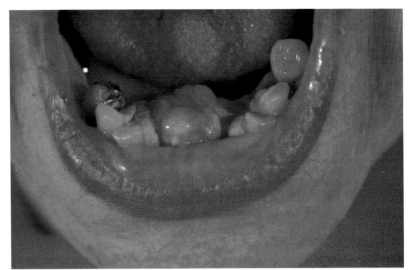

EPULIS. Female; *age* 62 years; *duration* 4 months; mouth; confirmed by biopsy.

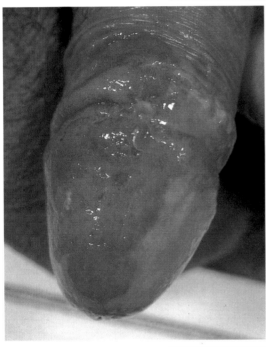

ERYTHROPLASIA OF QUEY-RAT. Male; *age* 61 years; *duration* 3 years; glans penis; confirmed by biopsy.

ERYTHROPLASIA OF QUEY-RAT. Male; *age* 64 years; *duration* 18 months; glans penis.

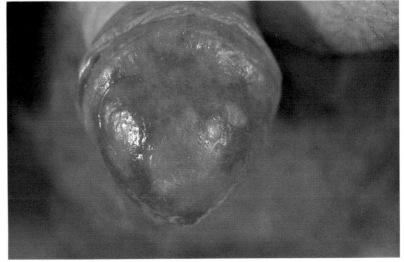

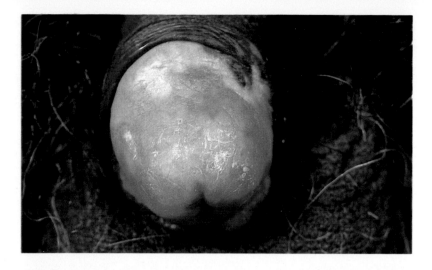

ERYTHROPLASIA OF QUEY-RAT. Male; *age* 43 years; *duration* 4 months; glans penis; confirmed by biopsy.

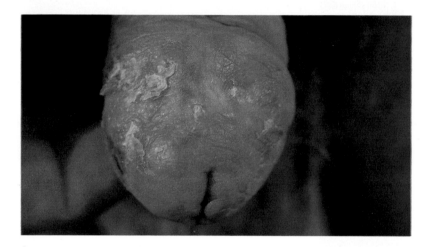

ERYTHROPLASIA OF QUEY-RAT. Male; *age* 48 years; *duration* 19 years; glans penis; confirmed by biopsy.

ERYTHROPLASIA OF QUEY-RAT. Male; *age* 58 years; *duration* 3 years; penis; con-firmed by biopsy.

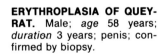

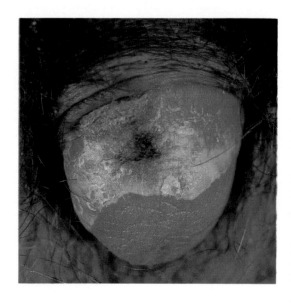

ERYTHROPLASIA OF QUEY-RAT. Male; glans penis, confirmed by biopsy.

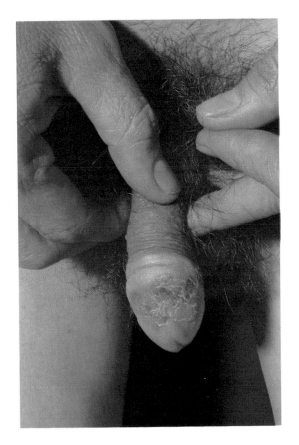

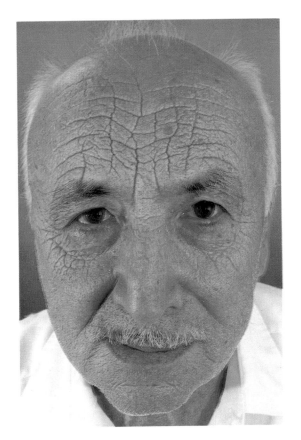

FAVRE-RACOUCHOT SYN-DROME. Male; *age* 68 years; *duration* years; forehead, malar area.

FAVRE-RACOUCHOT SYN-DROME. Male; *age* 68 years; *duration* years; forehead. (Patient also has basal-cell carcinoma on forehead.) (Same patient as in previous photograph.)

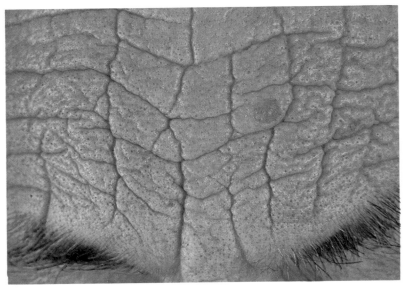

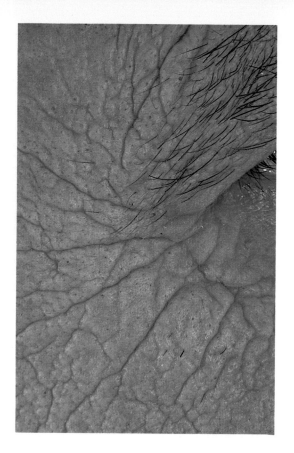

FAVRE-RACOUCHOT SYN-DROME. Male; *age* 68 years; *duration* years; periocular area. (Same patient as in previous photograph.)

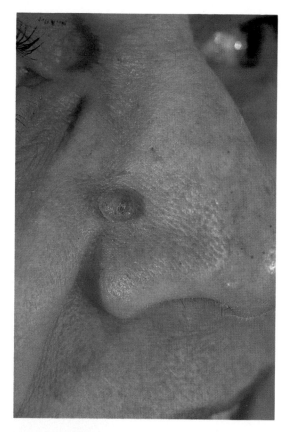

FIBROANGIOMA. Female; *age* 65 years; *duration* 3 years; nose; confirmed by biopsy.

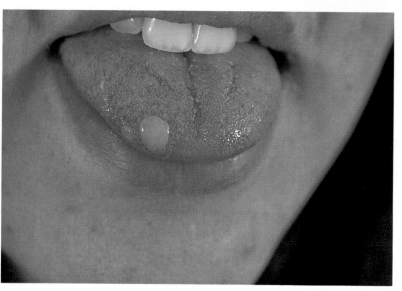

FIBROANGIOMA. Tongue.

FIBROANGIOMA. Female; *age* 3 years; finger; con-firmed by biopsy.

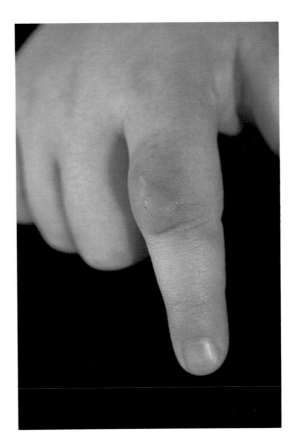

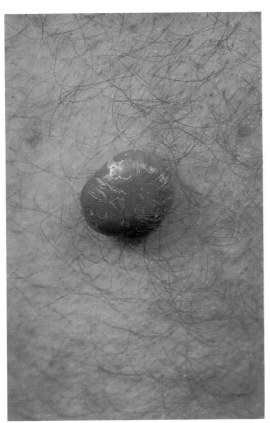

FIBROMA. Male; *age* 24 years; *duration* 6 years; thigh; confirmed by biopsy.

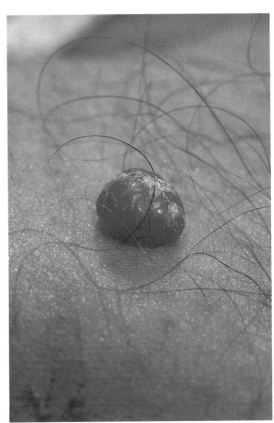

FIBROMA. Male; *age* 35 years; *duration* 3 years; arm; confirmed by biopsy.

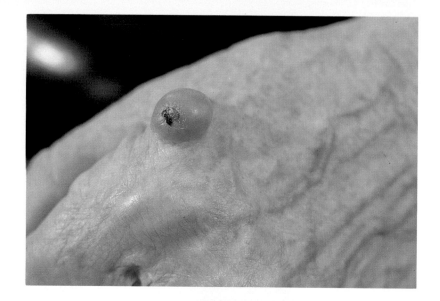

FIBROMA. Female; *age* 72 years; *duration* 20 years; hand.

FIBROMA. Female; *age* 31 years; *duration* 3 years; great toe; confirmed by biopsy.

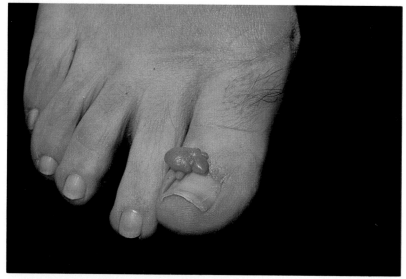

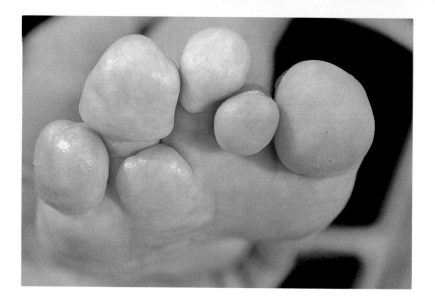

FIBROMA. Female; *age* 4 years; sole; confirmed by biopsy.

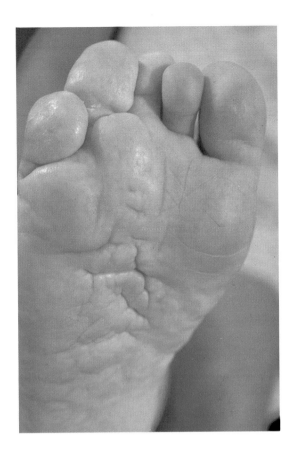

FIBROMA. Female; *age* 4 years; sole; confirmed by biopsy. (Same patient as in previous photograph.)

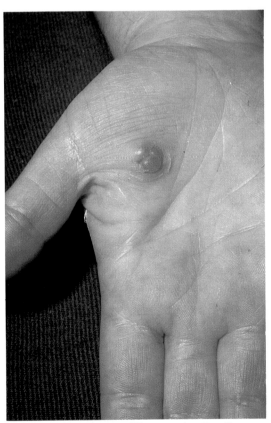

FIBROMA. Female; *age* 37 years; *duration* 5 years; palm; confirmed by biopsy.

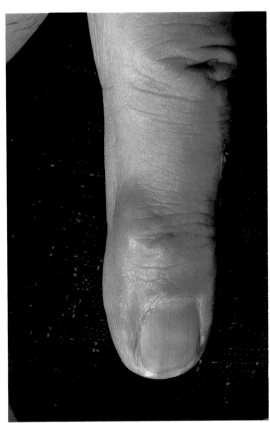

FIBROMA. Male; *age* 57 years; *duration* 4 years; index finger; confirmed by biopsy.

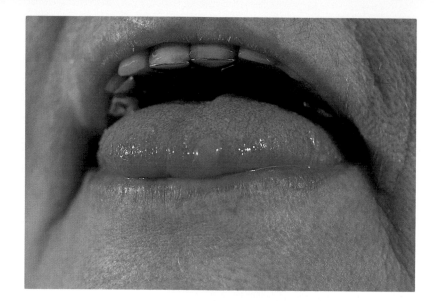

FIBROMA. Tongue.

FIBROMA. Female; *age* 61 years; *duration* 13 months; tongue; confirmed by biopsy.

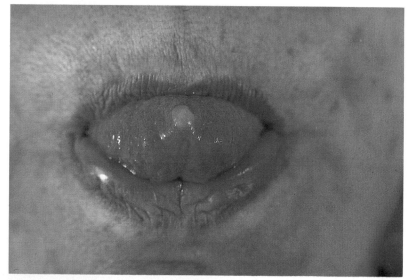

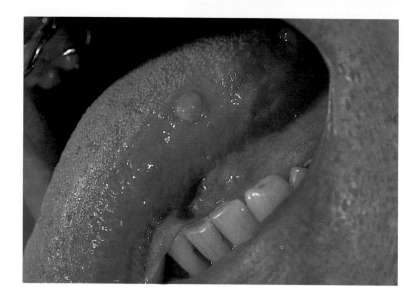

FIBROMA. Male; *age* 48 years; *duration* 13 months; tongue; confirmed by biopsy.

FIBROMAS. Female; *age* 44 years; tongue; confirmed by biopsy.

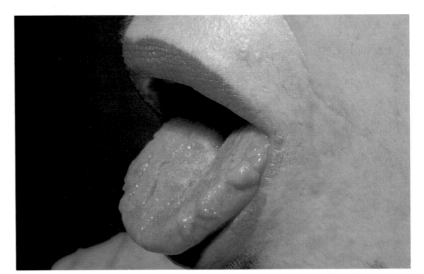

FIBROEPITHELIAL TUMOR (PINKUS). Male; *age* 65 years; *duration* 18 months; chest; confirmed by biopsy.

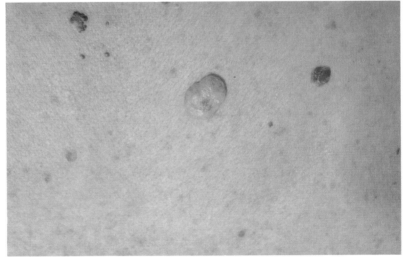

FIBROEPITHELIAL TUMOR (PINKUS). Male; *age* 68 years; *duration* 2 years; thigh; confirmed by biopsy.

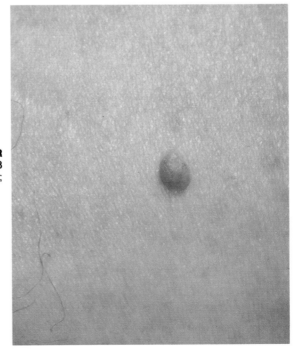

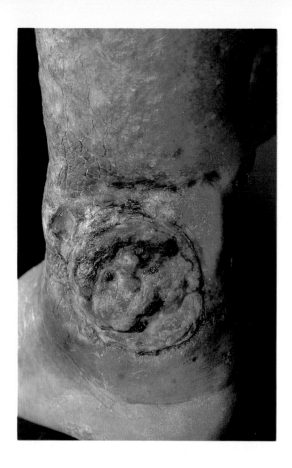

FIBROSARCOMA. Male; *age* 69 years; *duration* "years"; leg; confirmed by biopsy.

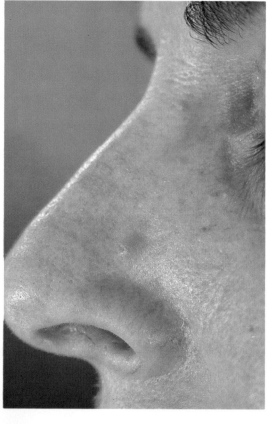

FIBROUS PAPULE OF THE NOSE. Female; *age* 40 years; *duration* 6 months; nose; confirmed by biopsy.

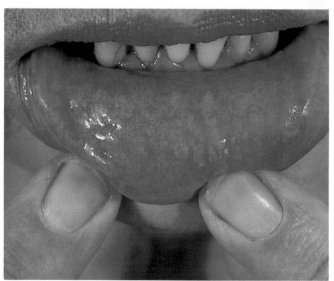

FORDYCE CONDITION. Female; *age* 57 years; labial mucosa; confirmed by biopsy.

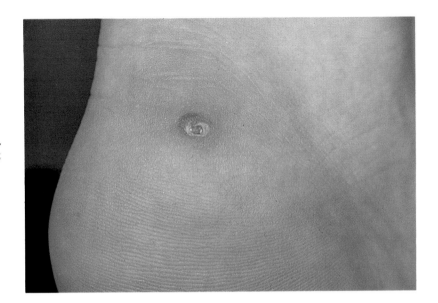

FOREIGN BODY GRANU-LOMA. Male; *age* 14 years; *duration* 7 months; heel.

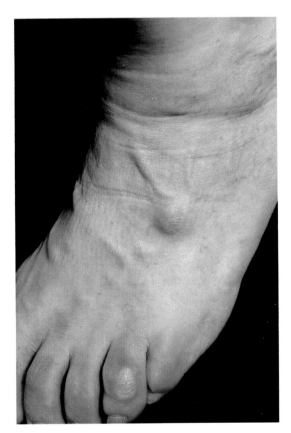

GANGLION. Male; *age* 48 years; *duration* 2 years; foot; confirmed by biopsy.

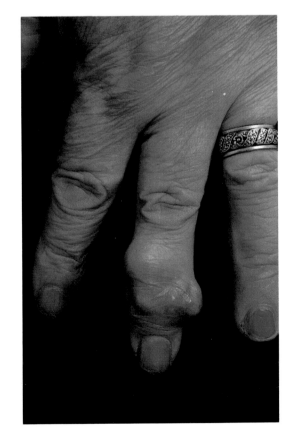

GIANT CELL TUMOR. Female; *age* 61 years; *duration* 4 years; finger; confirmed by biopsy.

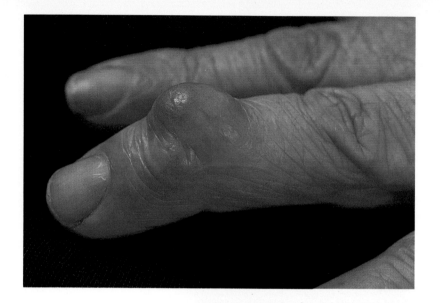

GIANT CELL TUMOR. Female; *age* 61 years; *duration* 4 years; finger; confirmed by biopsy. (Same patient as in previous photograph.)

GIANT CELL TUMOR. Female; *age* 54 years; *duration* 10 years; finger; confirmed by biopsy.

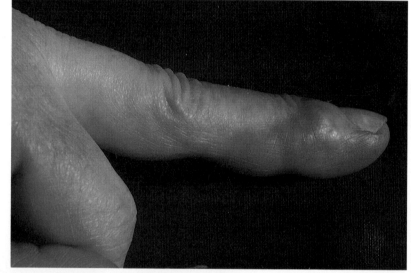

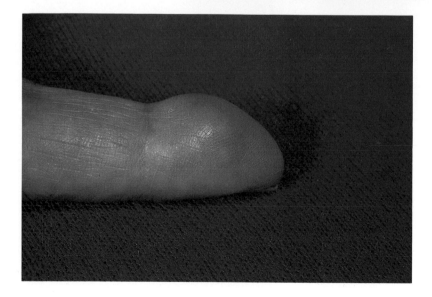

GIANT CELL TUMOR. Female; *age* 58 years; *duration* 13 months; index finger; confirmed by biopsy.

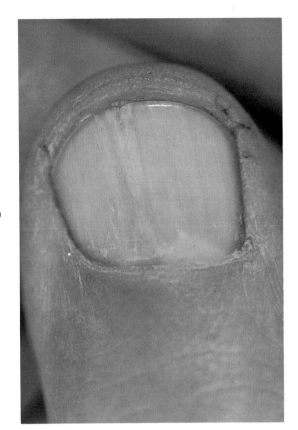

GLOMUS TUMOR.   Male; *age* 35 years; *duration* 10 years; proximal nail fold; confirmed by biopsy.

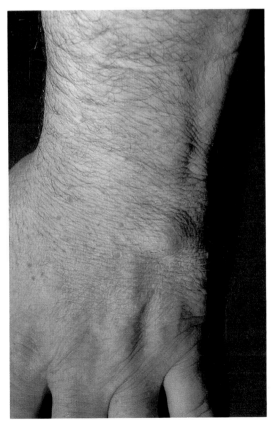

GLOMUS TUMOR.   Male; *age* 48 years; *duration* 10 years; hand; confirmed by biopsy.

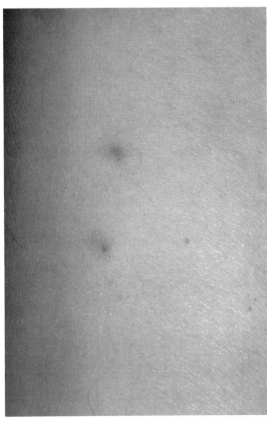

GLOMUS TUMORS.   Male; *age* 62 years; *duration* 4 months; arm; confirmed by biopsy.

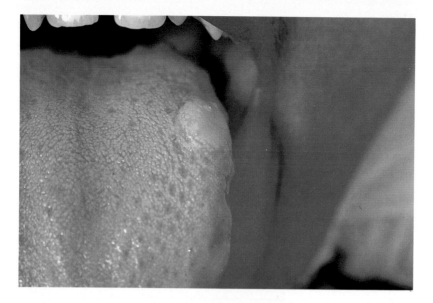

GRANULAR CELL SCHWAN-NOMA ("MYOBLASTOMA"). Female; *age* 29 years; *duration* 2 years; tongue; confirmed by biopsy.

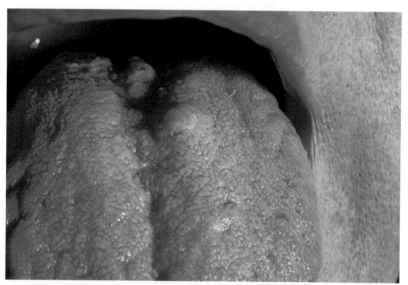

GRANULAR CELL SCHWAN-NOMA ("MYOBLASTOMA"). Male; *age* 54 years; tongue; confirmed by biopsy.

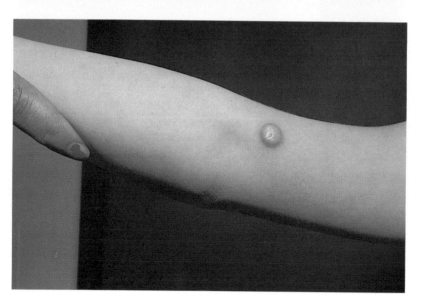

GRANULAR CELL SCHWAN-NOMA ("MYOBLASTOMA"). Male; *age* 4 years; *duration* 2 years; arm; confirmed by biopsy.

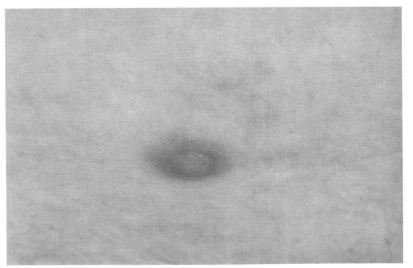

GRANULAR CELL SCHWAN-NOMA ("MYOBLASTOMA"). Female; *age* 76 years; *duration* 6 months; abdominal wall; confirmed by biopsy.

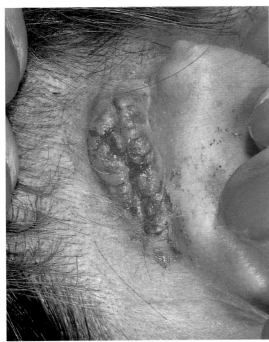

GRANULAR CELL SCHWAN-NOMA ("MYOBLASTOMA"). Female; *age* 47 years; behind ear; confirmed by biopsy.

GRANULOMA FACIALE. Male; *age* 60 years; *duration* 2 years; face; confirmed by biopsy.

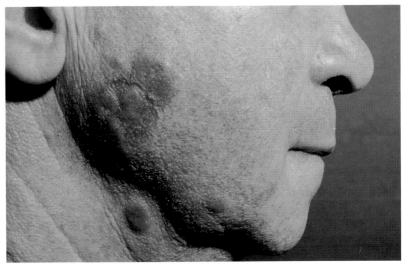

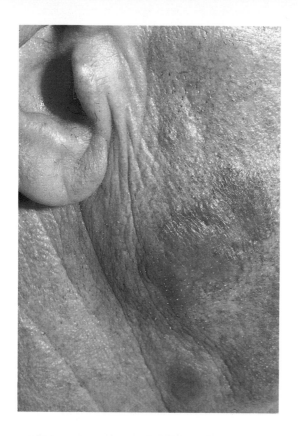

GRANULOMA FACIALE.
Male; *age* 60 years; *duration* 2 years; face; confirmed by biopsy. (Same patient as in previous photograph.)

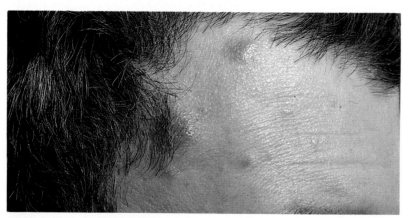

GRANULOMA FACIALE.
Male; *age* 60 years; *duration* 2 years; face; confirmed by biopsy. (Same patient as in previous photograph.)

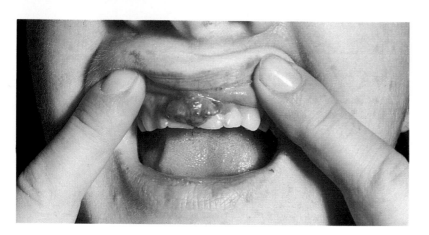

GRANULOMA TELANGIEC-TATICUM. Female; gingiva.

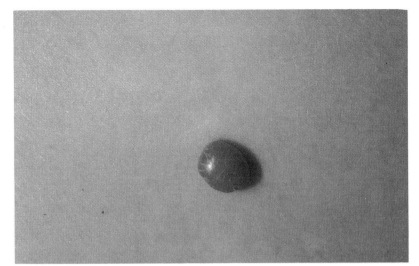

GRANULOMA TELANGIEC-TATICUM. Male; *age* 11 years; *duration* 18 months; back; confirmed by biopsy.

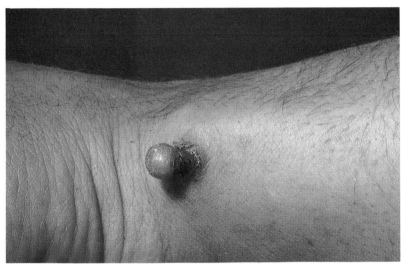

GRANULOMA TELANGIEC-TATICUM. Male; *age* 25 years; *duration* 3 years; wrist; confirmed by biopsy.

GRANULOMA TELANGIEC-TATICUM. Male; *age* 26 years; *duration* 7 months; trunk; confirmed by biopsy.

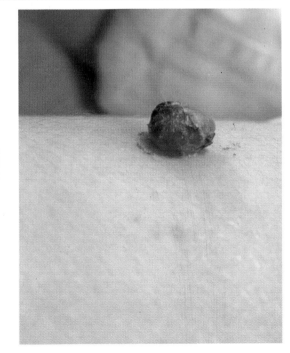

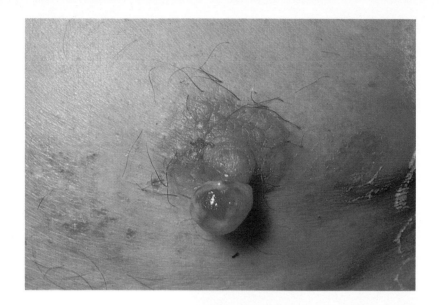

GRANULOMA TELANGIEC-TATICUM. Male; *age* 74 years; *duration* 8 days; nipple; confirmed by biopsy.

GRANULOMA TELANGIEC-TATICUM. Male; *age* 59 years; *duration* 7 months; forehead; confirmed by biopsy.

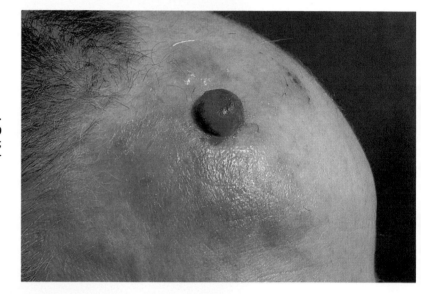

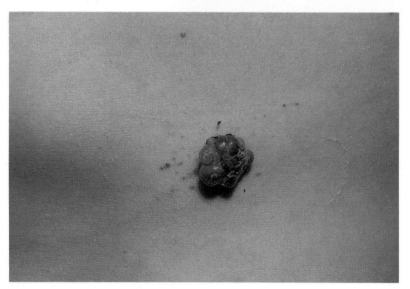

GRANULOMA TELANGIEC-TATICUM. Male; *age* 22 years; *duration* 4 months; abdominal wall; confirmed by biopsy.

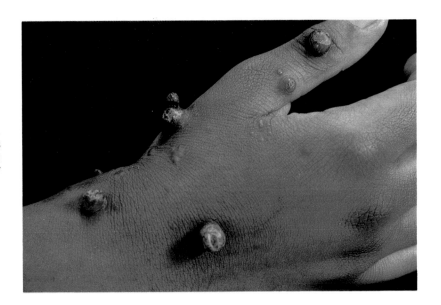

GRANULOMA TELANGIEC-TATICUM. Female; *age* 18 years; *duration* 13 months; wrist and hand; confirmed by biopsy.

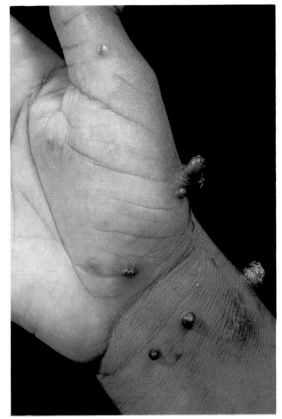

GRANULOMATA TELANGIECTATICA. Female; *age* 18 years; *duration* 13 months; wrist and hand; confirmed by biopsy. (Same patient as in previous photograph.)

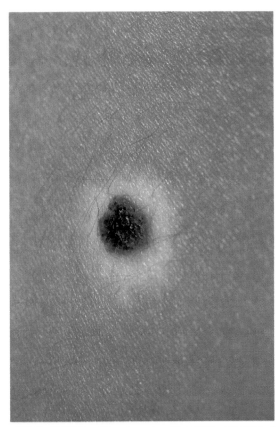

HALO NEVUS. Female; *age* 13 years; *duration* 4 months; back; confirmed by biopsy.

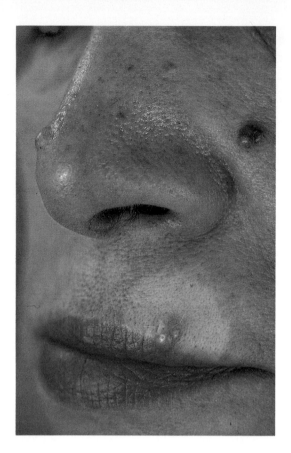

HALO NEVUS. Female; *age* 50 years; *duration* 4 years; nose.

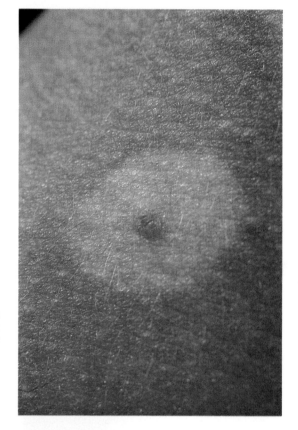

HALO NEVUS. Female; *age* 14 years; *duration* 4 months; upper trunk; confirmed by biopsy.

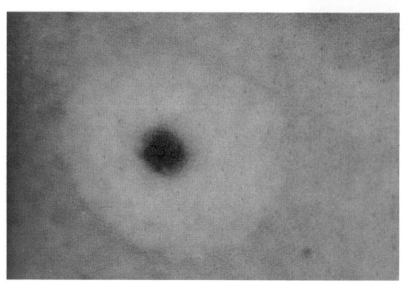

HALO NEVUS. Female; *age* 17 years; *duration* since birth; breast; confirmed by biopsy.

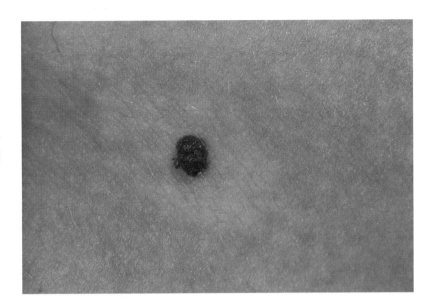

HALO NEVUS. Female; *age* 14 years; *duration* 4 months; arm, upper trunk; confirmed by biopsy.

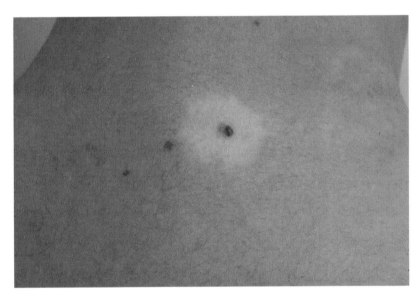

HALO NEVUS. Male; *age* 24 years; *duration* 7 years; neck; confirmed by biopsy.

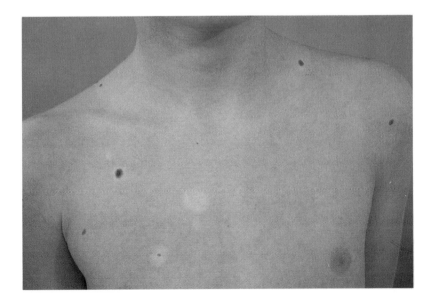

HALO NEVI. Male; *age* 11 years; trunk.

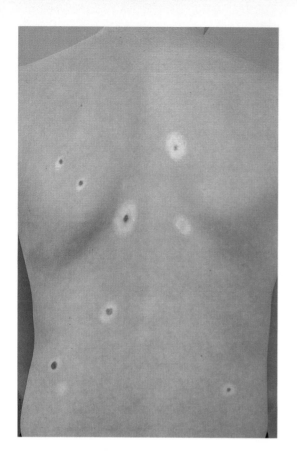

HALO NEVI. Male; *age* 12 years; back. (Same patient as in previous photograph.)

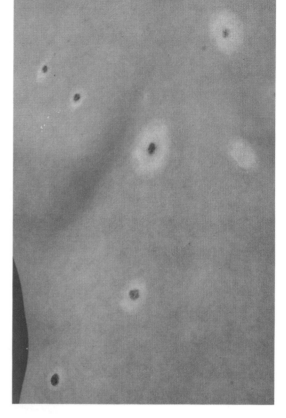

HALO NEVI. Male; *age* 12 years; chest, back. (Same patient as in previous photograph.)

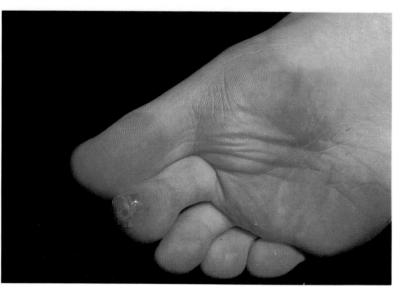

HEMANGIOENDOTHELIO-SARCOMA. Female; *age* 13 years; *duration* 6 months; second toe; confirmed by biopsy.

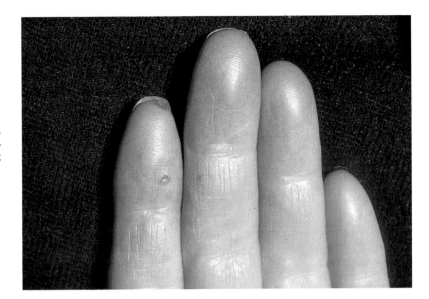

HEREDITARY HEMORRHAGIC TELANGIECTASIA. Female; *age* 68 years; fingers; confirmed by biopsy.

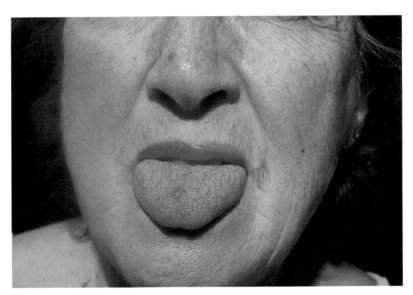

HEREDITARY HEMORRHAGIC TELANGIECTASIA. Female; *age* 68 years; tongue and face; confirmed by biopsy. (Same patient as in previous photograph.)

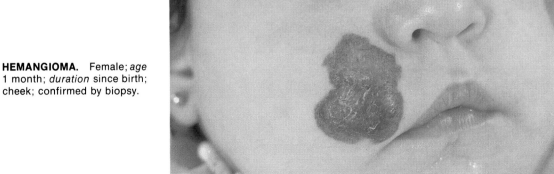

HEMANGIOMA. Female; *age* 1 month; *duration* since birth; cheek; confirmed by biopsy.

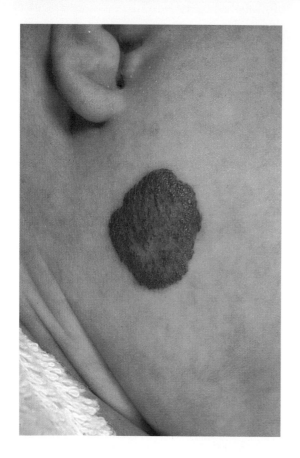

HEMANGIOMA. Female; *age* 3 months; *duration* since birth; cheek; confirmed by biopsy.

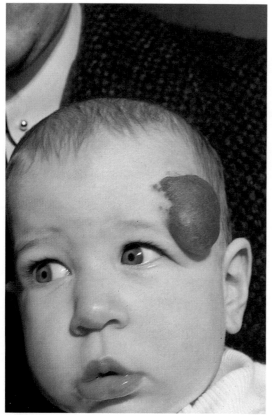

HEMANGIOMA. Female; *age* 3 months; *duration* since birth; forehead.

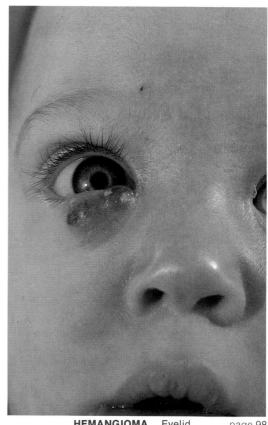

HEMANGIOMA. Eyelid. *page* 98

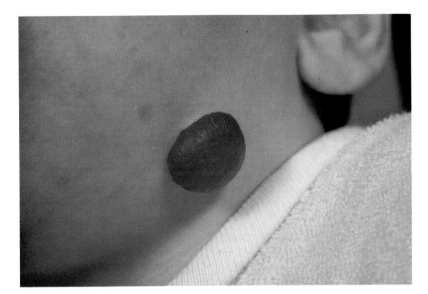

HEMANGIOMA. Male; *age* 7 months; *duration* since birth; cheek; confirmed by biopsy.

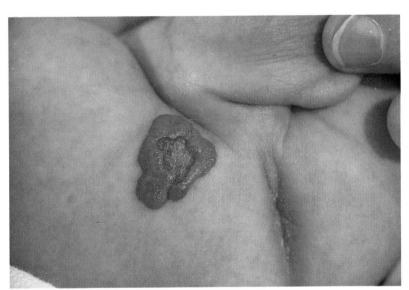

HEMANGIOMA. Male; thigh.

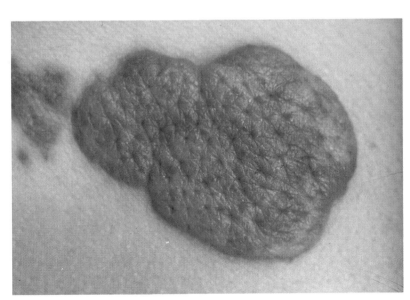

HEMANGIOMA. Male; *age* 3 years; *duration* since birth; back.

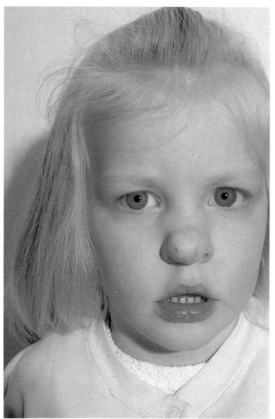

HEMANGIOMA.   Female; *age* 3 years; *duration* since age 1 month; nose.

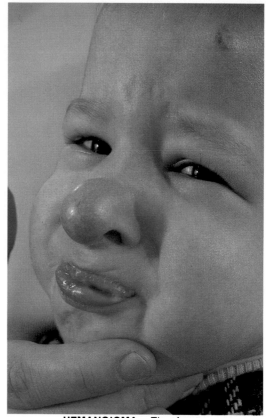

HEMANGIOMA.   Tip of nose.

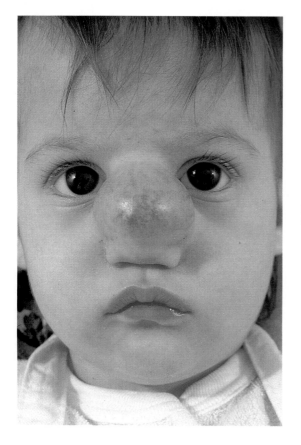

HEMANGIOMA.   Female; *age* 3 months; *duration* since birth; nose.

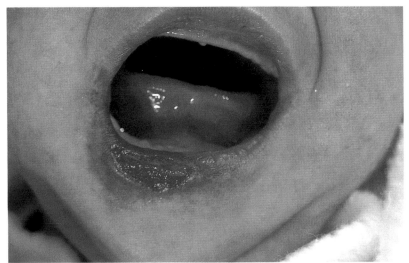

HEMANGIOMA. Female; *age* 2 months; *duration* began after birth; lower lip.

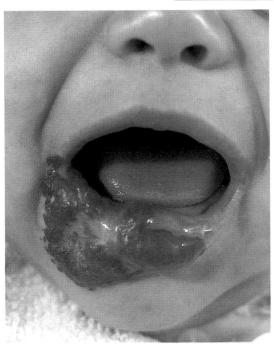

HEMANGIOMA. Female; *age* 6 months; *duration* began soon after birth; lower lip. (Same patient as in previous photograph.)

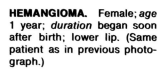

HEMANGIOMA. Female; *age* 1 year; *duration* began soon after birth; lower lip. (Same patient as in previous photograph.)

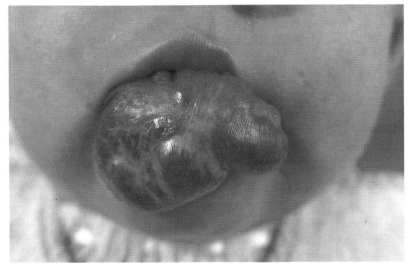

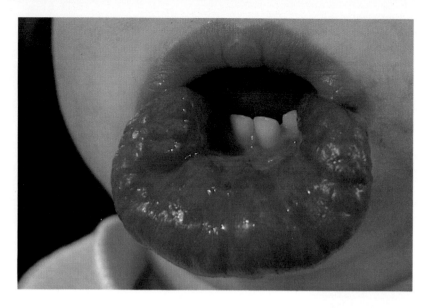

HEMANGIOMA. Female; *age* 14 months; *duration* 14 months; lower lip.

HEMANGIOMA. Male; *age* 4 months; *duration* 4 months; lip.

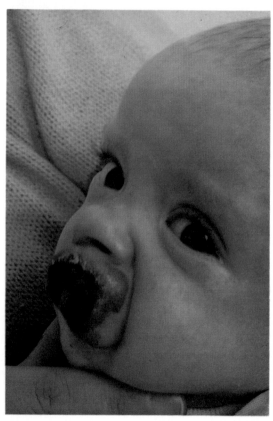

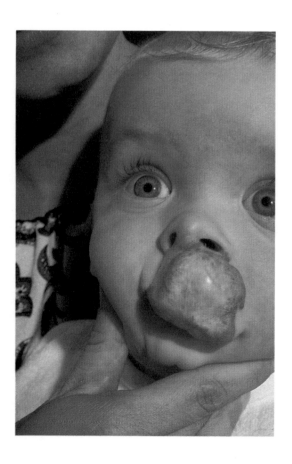

HEMANGIOMA. Male; *age* 2 years; *duration* 2 years; lip. (Same patient as in previous photograph.)

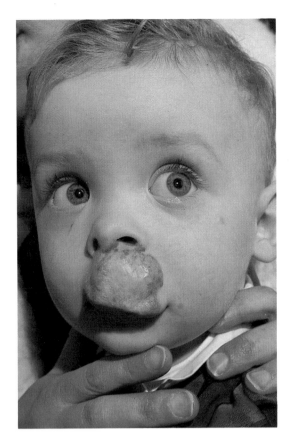

HEMANGIOMA.   Male; *age* 3 years; *duration* 3 years; lip. (Same patient as in previous photograph.)

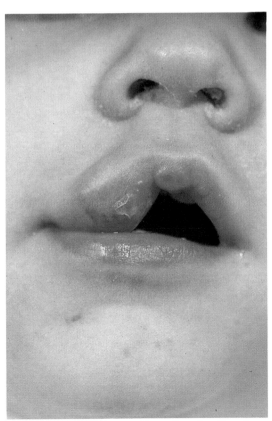

HEMANGIOMA.   Male; *age* 7 months; *duration* since birth; upper lip.

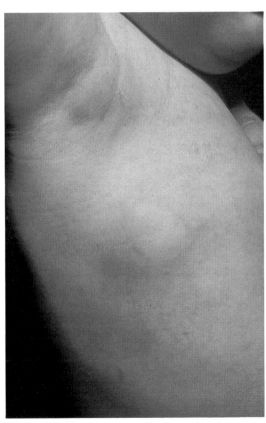

HEMANGIOMA.   Male; *age* 3 years; *duration* since birth; chest.

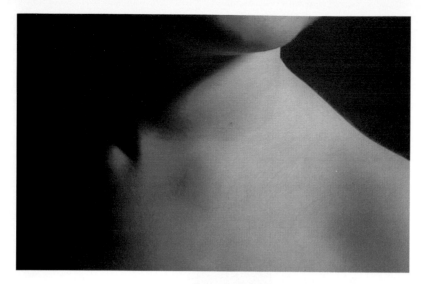

HEMANGIOMA.   Female; chest.

HEMANGIOMA.   Male; *age* 1;
duration 2 months; breast.

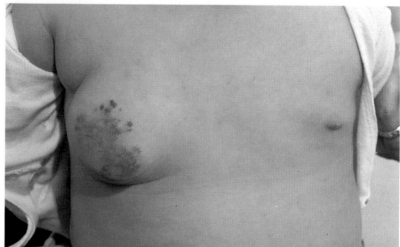

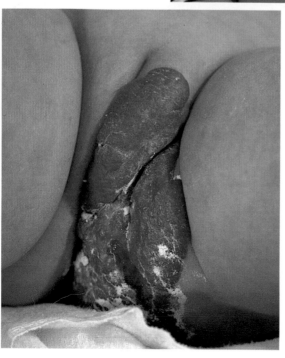

HEMANGIOMA.   Female;
vulva.

HEMANGIOMA. Female; *age* 4 months; *duration* since birth; arm and hand.

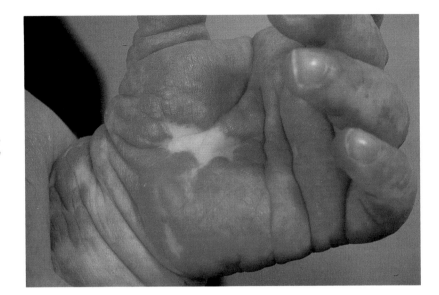

HEMANGIOMA. Female; *age* four-and-a-half years; upper extremity; confirmed by biopsy.

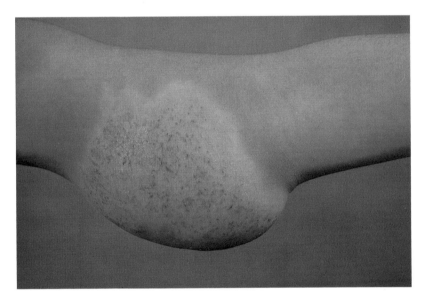

HEMANGIOMA. Female; *age* 6 years; *duration* 6 years; elbow area.

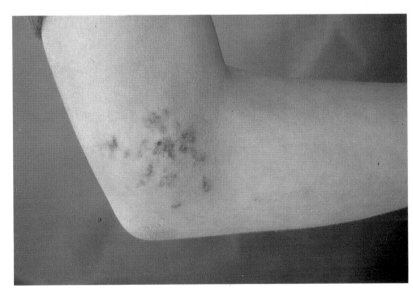

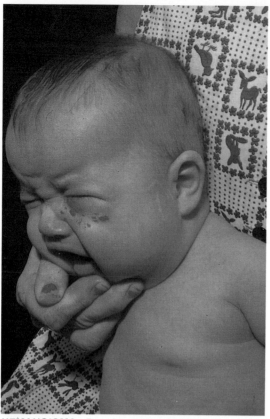

HEMANGIOMA. Female; *age* four-and-a-half months; *duration* four-and-a-half months; cheek.

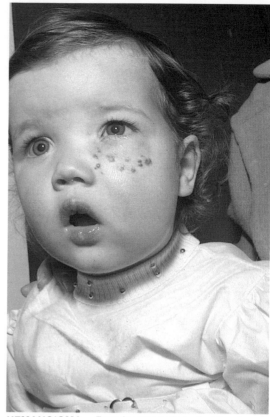

HEMANGIOMA. Female; *age* 1 year; *duration* 1 year; cheek. (Same patient as in previous photograph.)

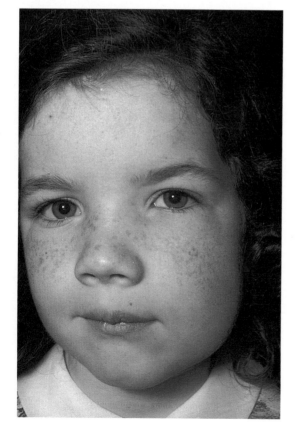

HEMANGIOMA. Female; *age* six-and-a-half years; *duration* six-and-a-half years; cheek. (Same patient as in previous photograph.)

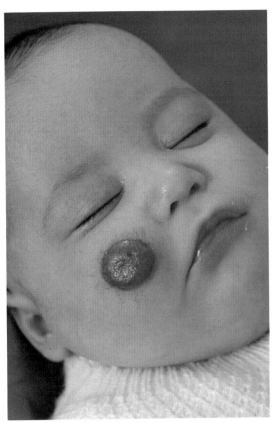

HEMANGIOMA. Female; *age* 2 months; *duration* 2 months; cheek.

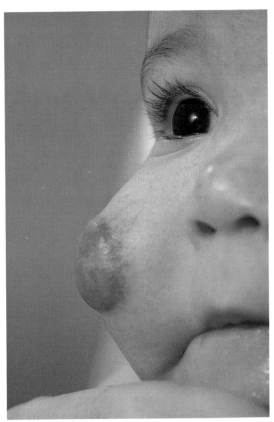

HEMANGIOMA. Female; *age* 5 months; *duration* 5 months; cheek. (Same patient as in previous photograph.)

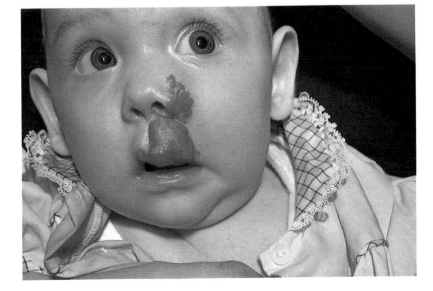

HEMANGIOMA. Female; *age* 4 months; *duration* 4 months; upper lip and nose; confirmed by biopsy.

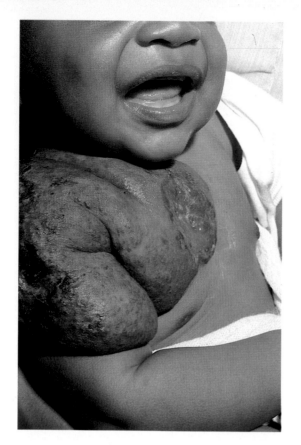

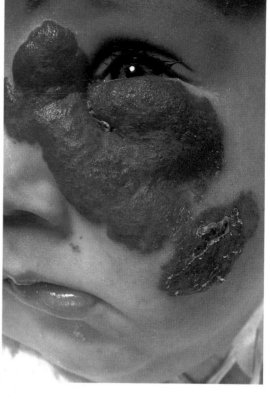

HEMANGIOMA. Male; *age* 3 months; *duration* 3 months; shoulder and chest.

HEMANGIOMA. Male; *age* infant; *duration* from one week after birth; cheek, nose, lower eyelid.

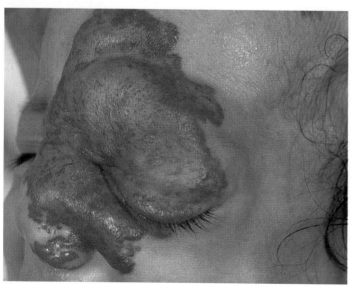

HEMANGIOMA. Female; *age* 4 months; *duration* 4 months; nose, eyelids.

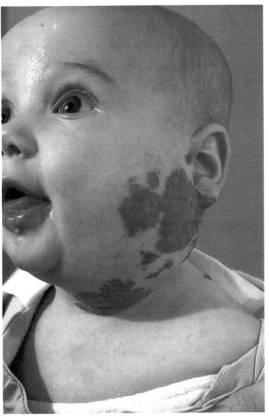

HEMANGIOMA. Male; *age* 5 weeks; *duration* 5 weeks; face and neck.

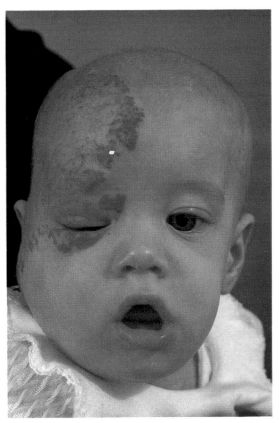

HEMANGIOMA. Female; *age* 4 months; *duration* 4 months; forehead, temple and eyelids.

HEMANGIOMA. Female; *age* 4 years; *duration* 4 years; forehead, temple, eyelids. (Same patient as in previous photograph.)

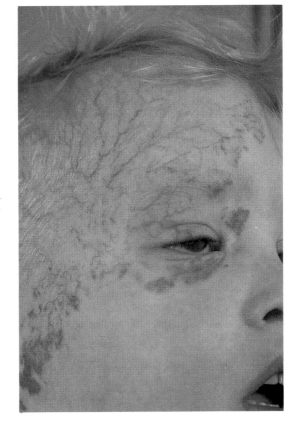

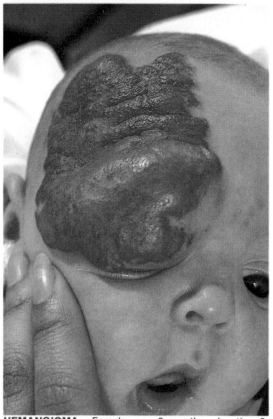

HEMANGIOMA. Female; *age* 2 months; *duration* 2 months; forehead and upper eyelid.

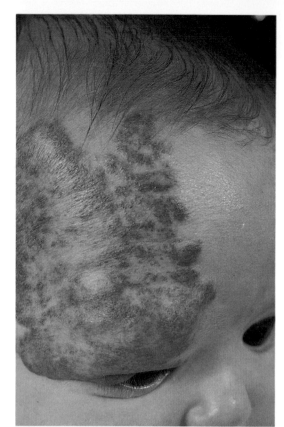

HEMANGIOMA. Female; *age* 6 months; *duration* 6 months; forehead and upper eyelid. (Same patient as in previous photograph.)

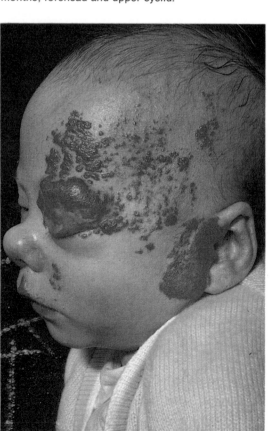

HEMANGIOMA. Male; *age* 6 months; *duration* 6 months; forehead, temple, upper eyelid, preauricular area.

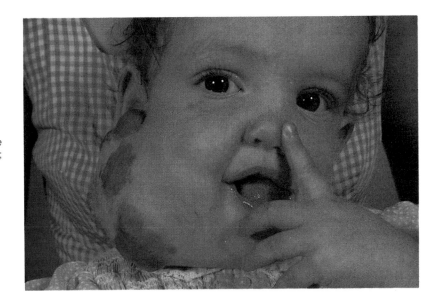

HEMANGIOMA. Female; *age* 4 months; *duration* 4 months; cheek and neck.

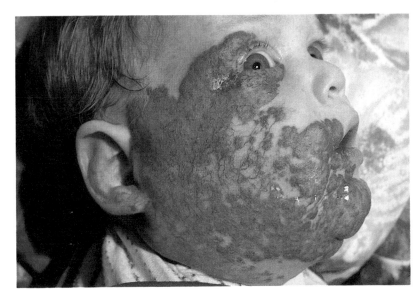

HEMANGIOMA. Female; *age* 4 months; face.

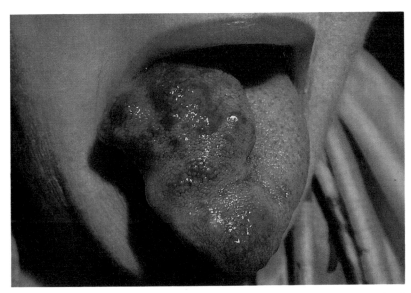

HEMANGIOMA. Female; *age* adult; *duration* life; tongue.

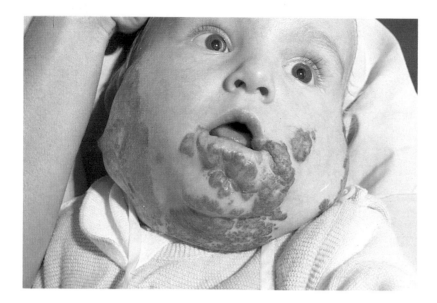

HEMANGIOMA. Male; *age* 11 weeks; *duration* 11 weeks; face and neck.

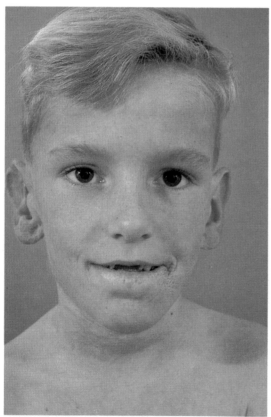

HEMANGIOMA. Male; *age* 6 years; *duration* 6 years; face and neck. (Same patient as in previous photograph.)

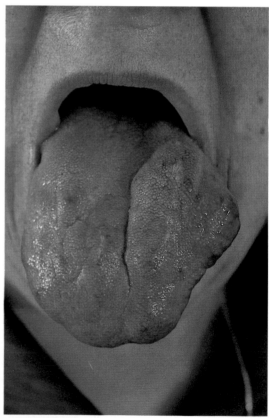

HEMANGIOMA. Female; *age* 55 years; *duration* 45 years; tongue; confirmed by biopsy.

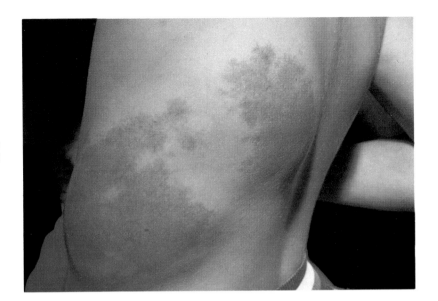

HEMANGIOMA. Female; *age* 4 years; *duration* 4 years; flank.

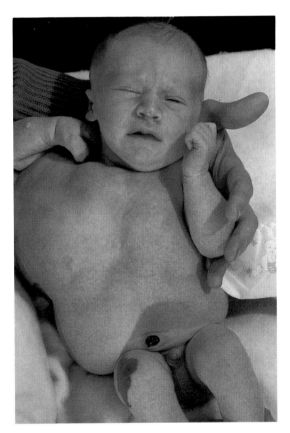

HEMANGIOMA. Male; *age* 2 weeks; chest and knee; confirmed by biopsy.

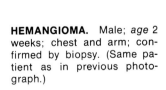

HEMANGIOMA. Male; *age* 2 weeks; chest and arm; confirmed by biopsy. (Same patient as in previous photograph.)

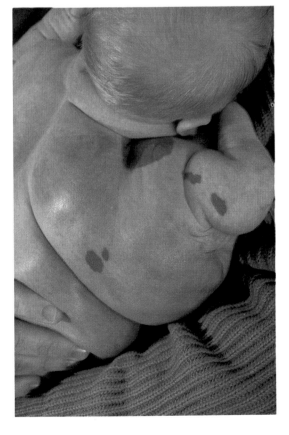

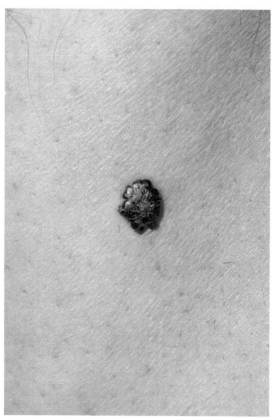

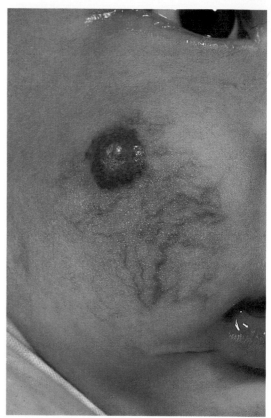

HEMANGIOMA. Male; *age* 30 years; *duration* 30 years; knee; confirmed by biopsy.

HEMANGIOMA, STRAWBERRY AND CAVERNOUS. Female; *age* 8 months.

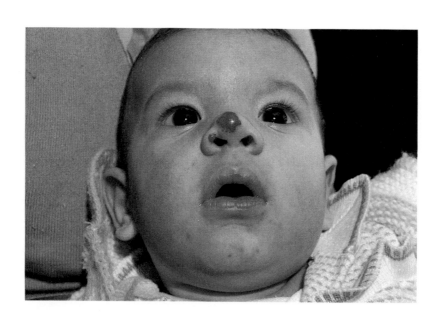

HEMANGIOMA, STRAW-BERRY. Male; *age* 3 months; *duration* 1 month; nose.

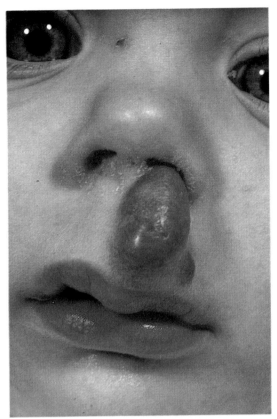

HEMANGIOMA, STRAWBERRY AND CAVERNOUS.
Upper lip.

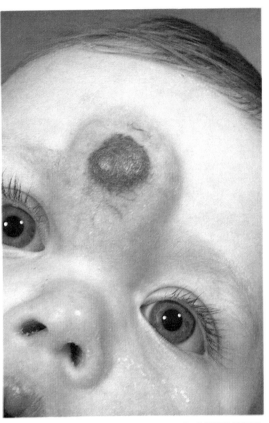

HEMANGIOMA, STRAWBERRY AND CAVERNOUS.
Female; *age* 5 months; *duration* since birth; forehead.

**HEMANGIOMA, STRAW-
BERRY AND CAVERNOUS.**
Female; *age* 7 months; *dura-
tion* 6 months; scalp.

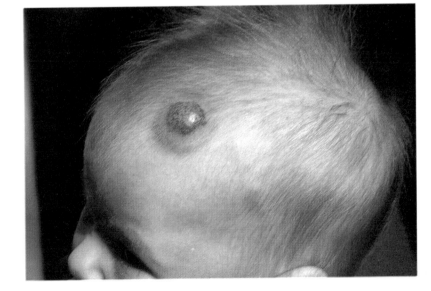

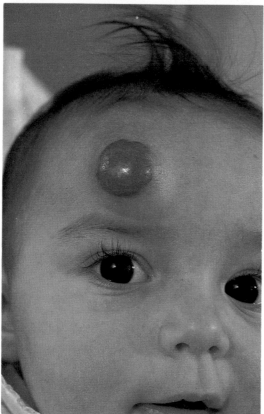

HEMANGIOMA, STRAWBERRY AND CAVERNOUS.
Female; *age* 5 months; *duration* since birth; forehead.

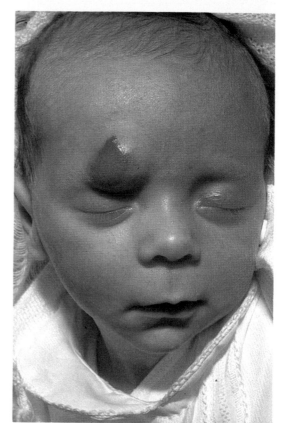

HEMANGIOMA, STRAWBERRY AND CAVERNOUS.
Male; *age* 8 weeks; *duration* since birth; forehead.

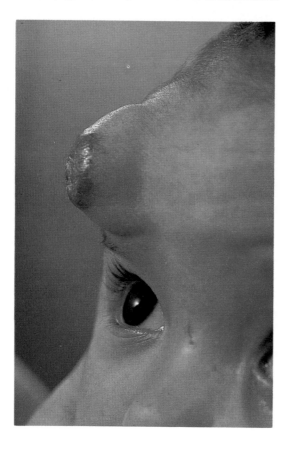

HEMANGIOMA, STRAWBERRY AND CAVERNOUS.
Female; *age* 5 months; *duration* since birth; forehead.
(Same patient as in photo above.)

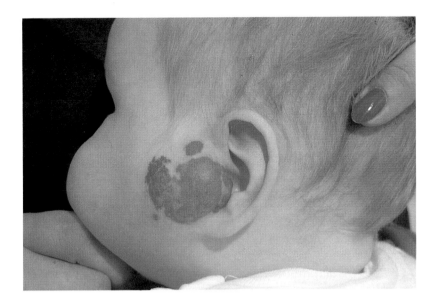

HEMANGIOMA, STRAW-BERRY AND CAVERNOUS. Male; *age* 8 months; *duration* since birth; preauricular area.

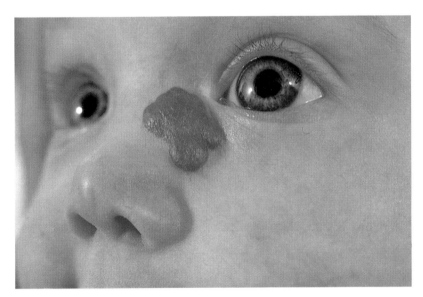

HEMANGIOMA, STRAW-BERRY. Female; *age* 5 months; *duration* since birth; nose.

HEMANGIOMA, STRAW-BERRY. Female; *age* 6 months; *duration* since birth; back.

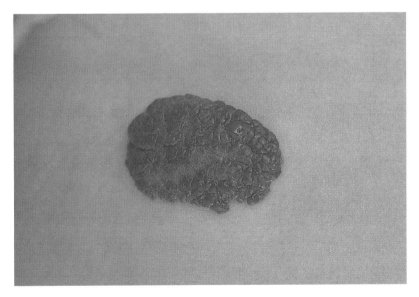

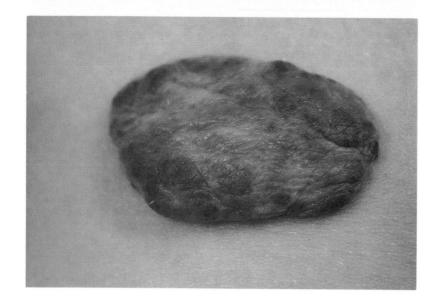

**HEMANGIOMA, STRAW-
BERRY.** Male; *age* 8 months;
duration 6 months; back.

**HEMANGIOMA, STRAW-
BERRY.** Female; *age* 4
months; *duration* since birth;
eyelids and paranasal area.

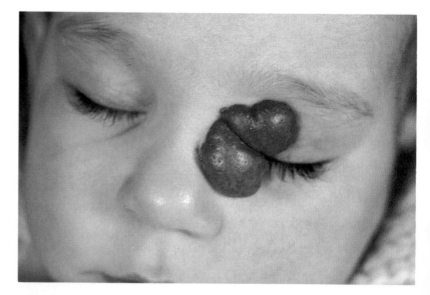

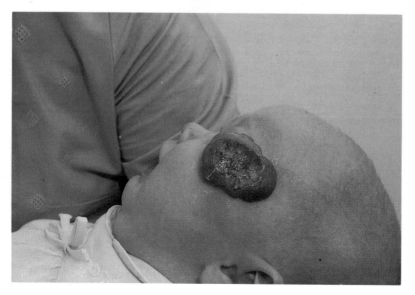

**HEMANGIOMA, STRAW-
BERRY.** Female; *age* 3
months; *duration* since birth;
malar area and temple.

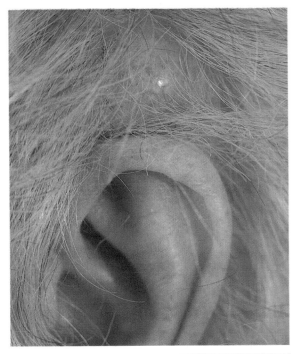

HIDRADENOMA PAPILLI-FERUM. Scalp; confirmed by biopsy.

HIDROCYSTOMA. Female; *age* 37 years; *duration* 7 months; nose; confirmed by biopsy.

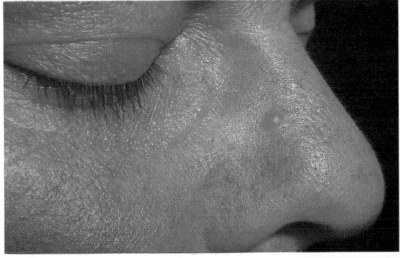

HIDROCYSTOMAS. Female; *age* 70 years; *duration* 2 years; cheek; confirmed by biopsy.

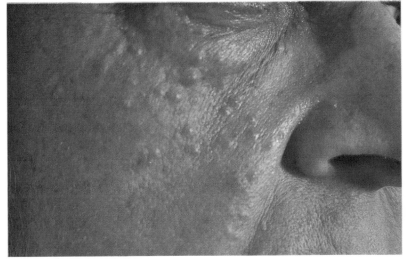

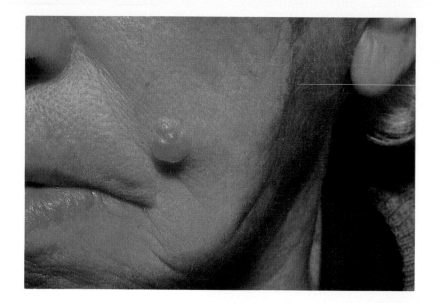

HIDROCYSTOMA. Female; *age* 77 years; *duration* 5 years; cheek; confirmed by biopsy.

INVERTED FOLLICULAR KERATOSIS. Male; *age* 58 years; *duration* 1 year; nose; confirmed by biopsy.

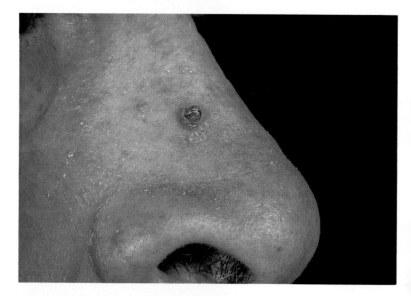

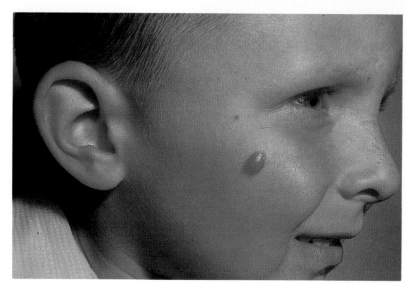

JUVENILE XANTHOGRANU-LOMA. Male; *age* 7 years; *duration* 4 years; cheek; confirmed by biopsy.

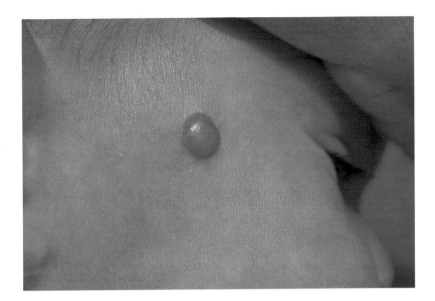

**JUVENILE XANTHOGRANU-
LOMA.** Female; *age* 6 months; *duration* 4 months; cheek; confirmed by biopsy.

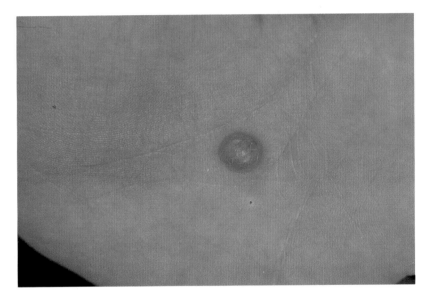

**JUVENILE XANTHOGRANU-
LOMA.** Male; *age* 9 years; *duration* 2 years; palm; confirmed by biopsy.

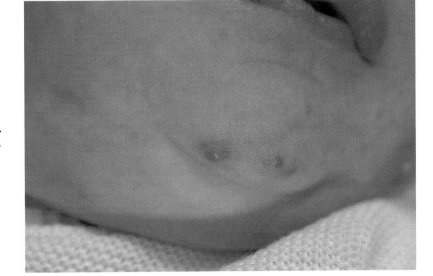

**JUVENILE XANTHOGRANU-
LOMA.** Male; infant; chin.

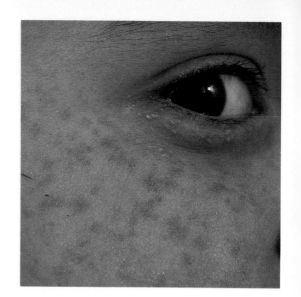

JUVENILE XANTHOGRANU-LOMA. Male; *age* 4 years; *duration* 9 months; face.

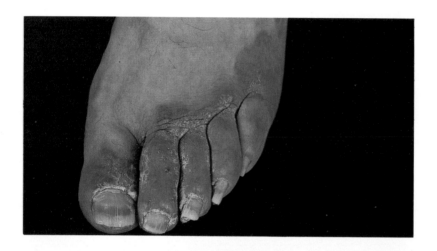

KAPOSI'S SARCOMA. Male; *age* 68 years; *duration* 2 years; foot; confirmed by biopsy.

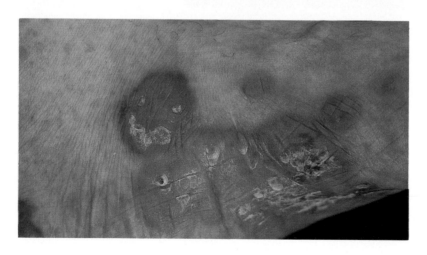

KAPOSI'S SARCOMA. Male; *age* 68 years; *duration* 2 years; foot; confirmed by biopsy. (Same patient as in previous photograph.)

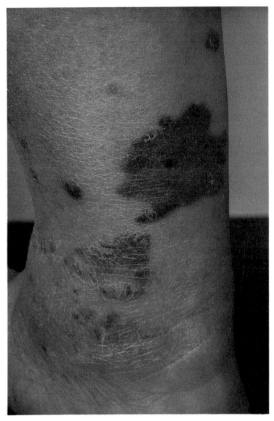

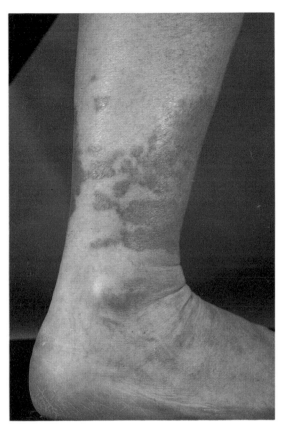

KAPOSI'S SARCOMA. Female; *age* 66 years; *duration* 9 years; leg and ankle; confirmed by biopsy.

KAPOSI'S SARCOMA. Female; *age* 59 years; *duration* 15 years; leg; confirmed by biopsy.

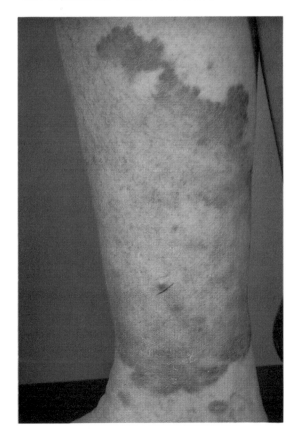

KAPOSI'S SARCOMA. Female; *age* 59 years; *duration* 15 years; leg; confirmed by biopsy. (Same patient as in previous photograph.)

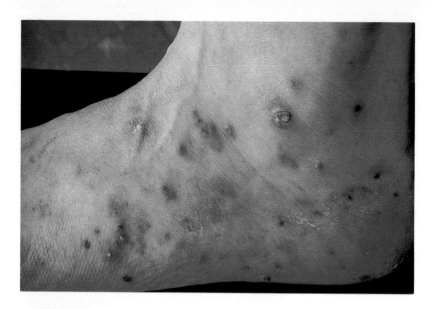

KAPOSI'S SARCOMA. Male; *age* 51 years; *duration* 5 years; foot; confirmed by biopsy.

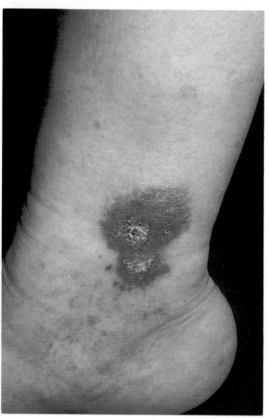

KAPOSI'S SARCOMA. Female; *age* 59 years; *duration* 7 years; ankle; confirmed by biopsy.

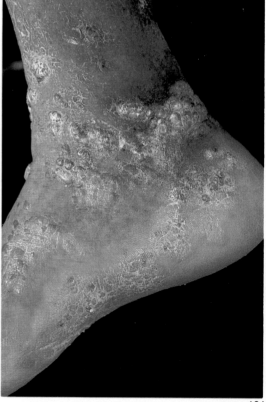

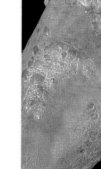

KAPOSI'S SARCOMA. Female; *age* 83 years; foot and ankle; confirmed by biopsy.

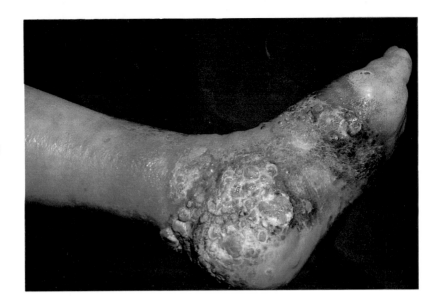

KAPOSI'S SARCOMA. Foot and leg.

KAPOSI'S SARCOMA. Male; leg.

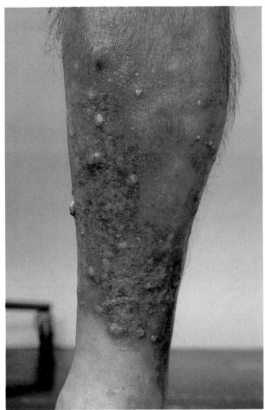
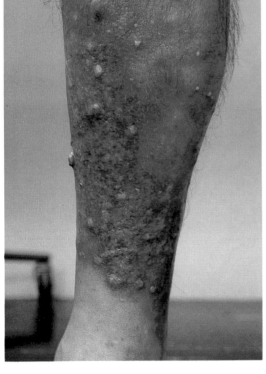
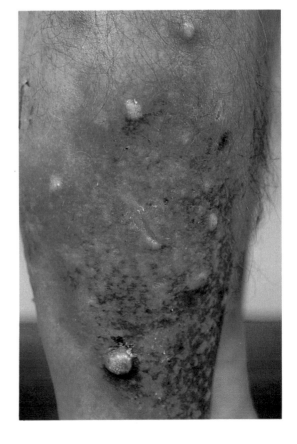

KAPOSI'S SARCOMA. Male; leg. (Same patient as in previous photograph.)

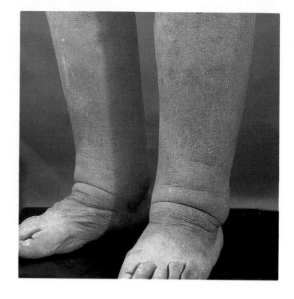

KAPOSI'S SARCOMA. Female; *age* 71 years; *duration* 9 months; legs; confirmed by biopsy.

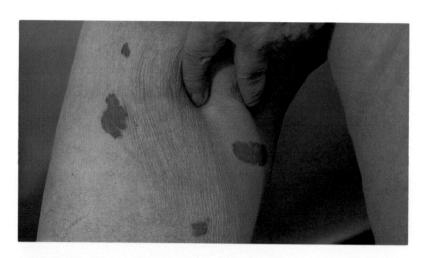

KAPOSI'S SARCOMA. Female; *age* 68 years; thigh.

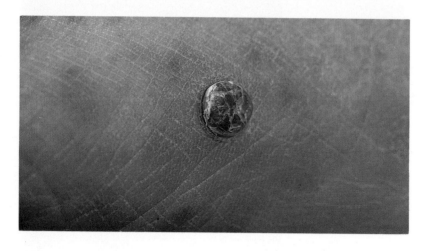

KAPOSI'S SARCOMA. Male; *age* 68 years; *duration* 2 years; foot; confirmed by biopsy.

KAPOSI'S SARCOMA. Female; *age* 62 years; *duration* 4 years; sole.

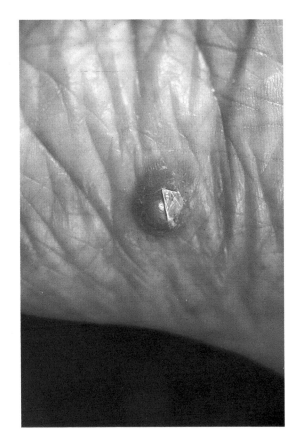

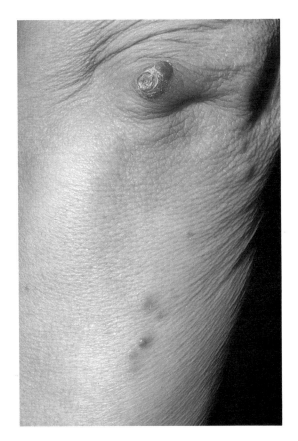

KAPOSI'S SARCOMA. Male; *age* 56 years; *duration* 12 years; elbow; confirmed by biopsy.

KAPOSI'S SARCOMA. Male; *age* 52 years; *duration* 1 year; hard palate.

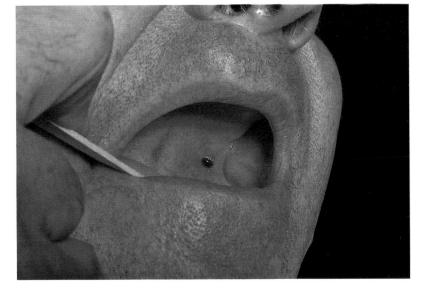

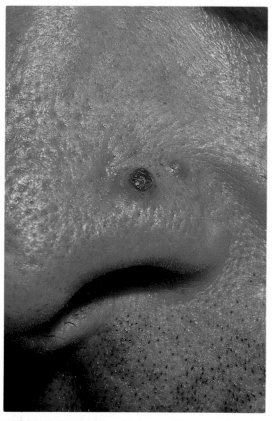

KAPOSI'S SARCOMA. Male; *age* 60 years; *duration* 3 months; nose; confirmed by biopsy.

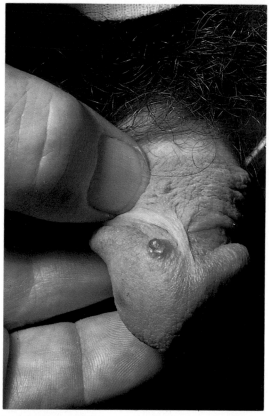

KAPOSI'S SARCOMA. Male; *age* 47 years; *duration* 2 weeks; penis; confirmed by biopsy.

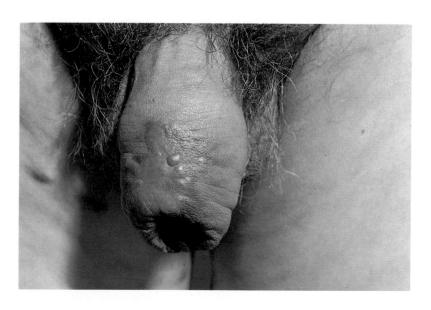

KAPOSI'S SARCOMA. Male; *age* 66 years; *duration* 1 year; penis; confirmed by biopsy.

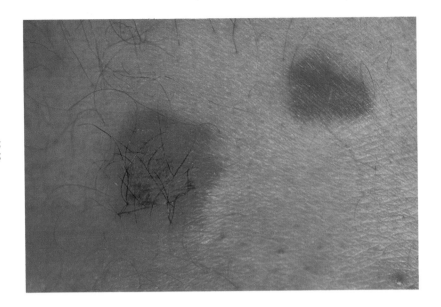

KAPOSI'S SARCOMA. Male; *age* 64 years; *duration* 9 years; leg; confirmed by biopsy.

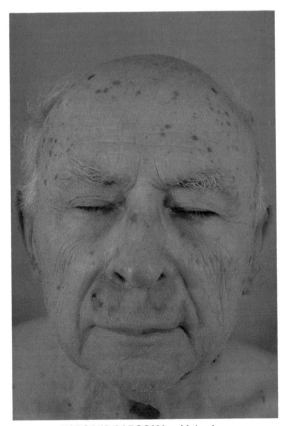

KAPOSI'S SARCOMA. Male; face.

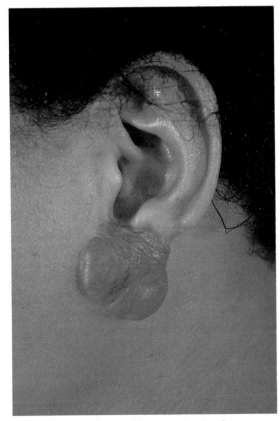

KELOID. Female; *age* 29 years; *duration* 9 years; ear; confirmed by biopsy.

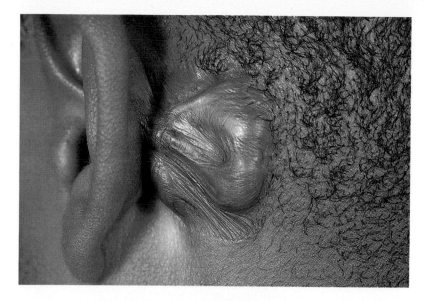

KELOID. Male; *age* 24 years; *duration* 5 years; retroauricular area; confirmed by biopsy.

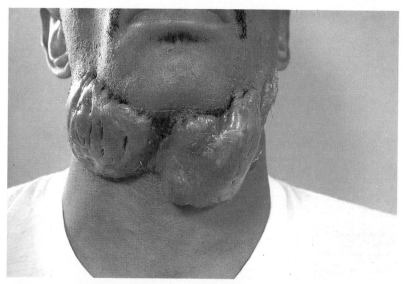

KELOID. Male; *age* 34 years; *duration* 8 years; neck.

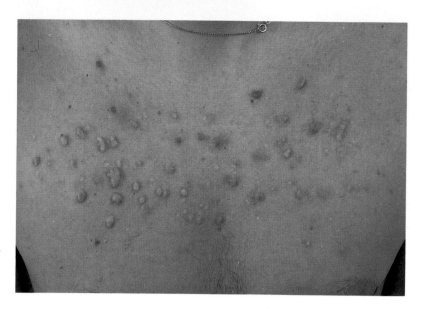

KELOIDS. Male; *age* 17 years; *duration* 8 years; chest.

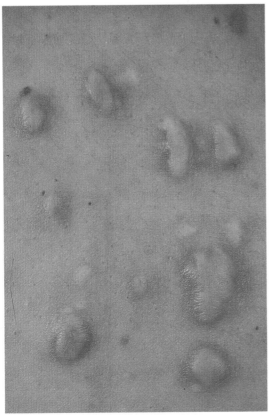

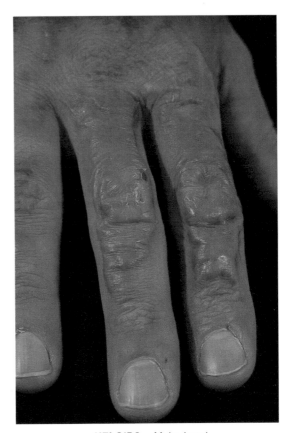

KELOIDS. Male; *age* 17 years; *duration* 8 years; chest. (Same patient as in previous photograph.)

KELOIDS. Male; hand.

KELOIDS. Male; *age* 14 years; *duration* 2 years; back.

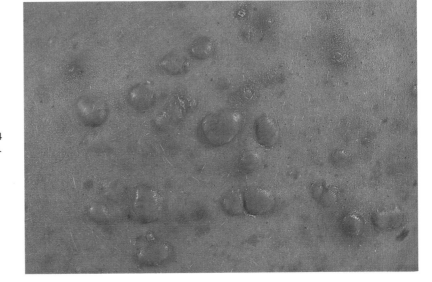

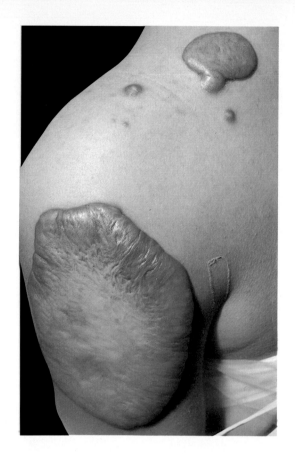

KELOIDS. Female; *age* 19 years; *duration* 13 years; shoulder and deltoid area.

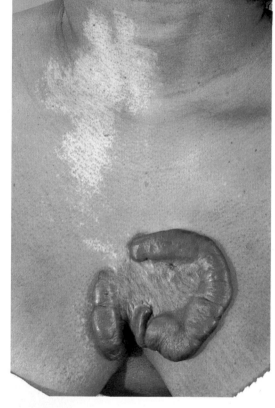

KELOID. Female; *age* 44 years; *duration* 12 years; chest; confirmed by biopsy.

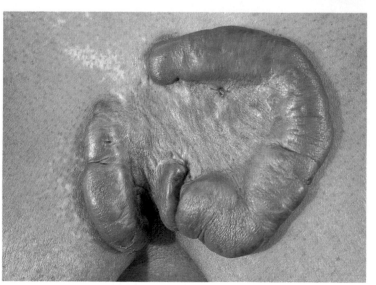

KELOID. Female; *age* 44 years; *duration* 12 years; chest; confirmed by biopsy. (Same patient as in previous photograph.)

KELOID. Male; *duration* 1 year; shoulder, back.

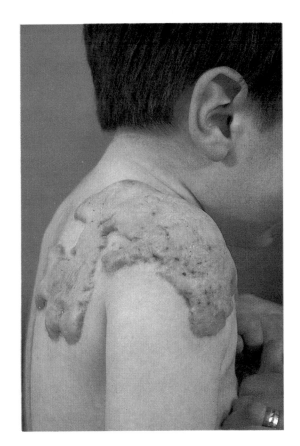

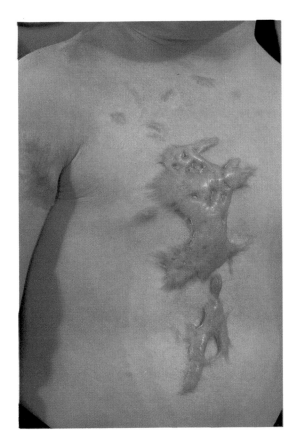

KELOIDS. Male; *age* 3 years; *duration* 7 months; chest and arm.

KELOID. Male; *age* 4 years; *duration* 3 months; penis.

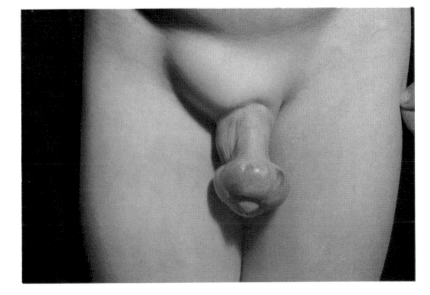

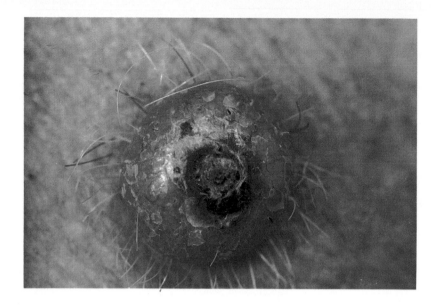

KERATOACANTHOMA. Male; *age* 84 years; *duration* 4 months; neck; confirmed by biopsy.

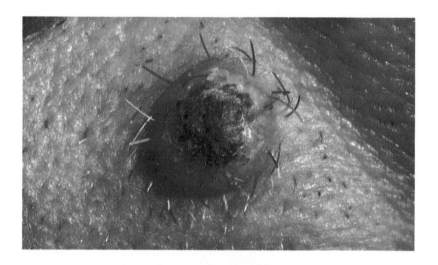

KERATOACANTHOMA. Face.

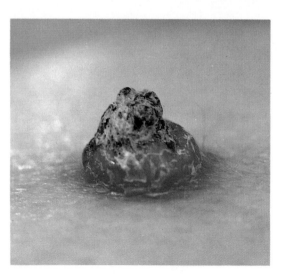

KERATOACANTHOMA. Female; *age* 61 years; *duration* 1 month; back; confirmed by biopsy.

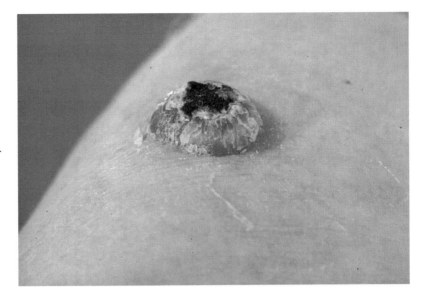

KERATOACANTHOMA. Shoulder.

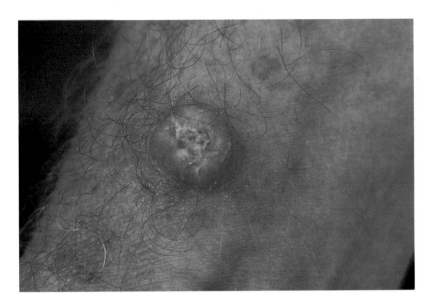

KERATOACANTHOMA. Male; *age* 63 years; *duration* 10 months; forearm; confirmed by biopsy.

KERATOACANTHOMA. Male; paranasal area; confirmed by biopsy.

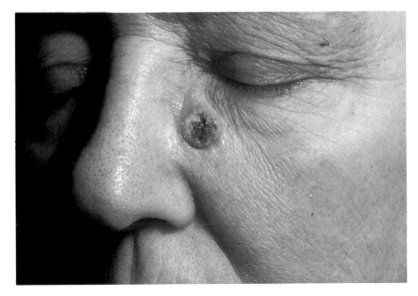

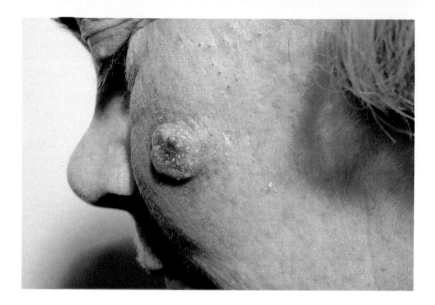

KERATOACANTHOMA. Female; *duration* 6 months; cheek; confirmed by biopsy.

KERATOACANTHOMA. Female; *age* 58 years; *duration* 4 months; upper lip; confirmed by biopsy.

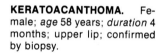
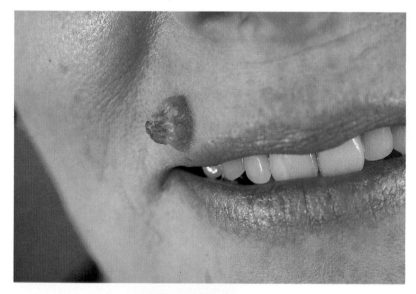

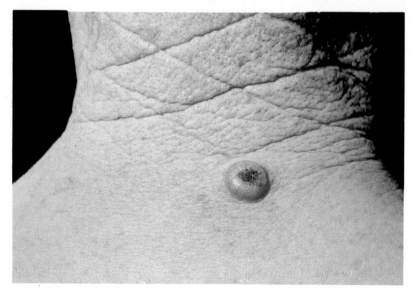

KERATOACANTHOMA. Male; neck; confirmed by biopsy.

KERATOACANTHOMA. Male; *age* 70 years; *duration* 3 months; scalp; confirmed by biopsy.

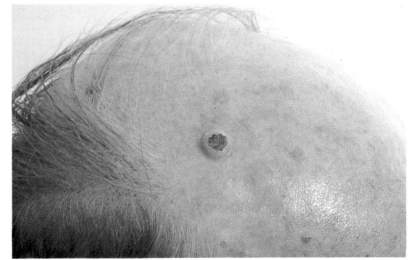

KERATOACANTHOMA. Male; forehead; confirmed by biopsy.

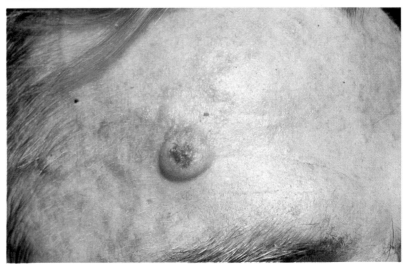

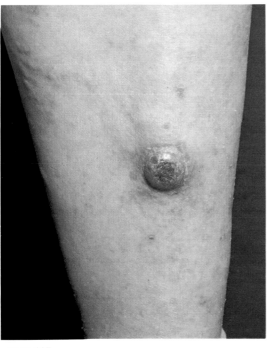

KERATOACANTHOMA. Female; *age* 63 years; *duration* 4 months; leg; confirmed by biopsy.

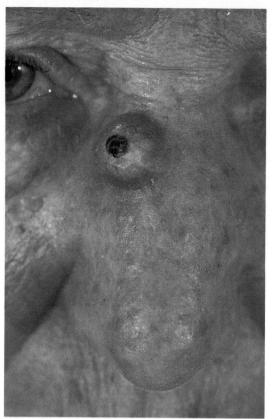

KERATOACANTHOMA. Female; nose; confirmed by biopsy.

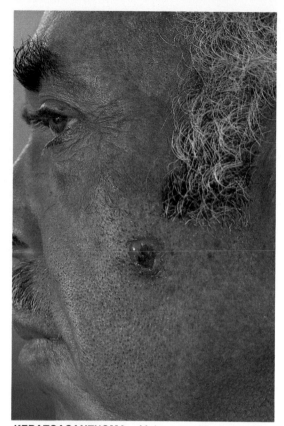

KERATOACANTHOMA. Male; *age* 68 years; *duration* 3 months; cheek.

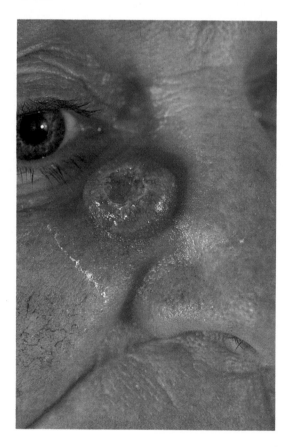

KERATOACANTHOMA. Female; *age* 54 years; *duration* 5 weeks; paranasal area; confirmed by biopsy.

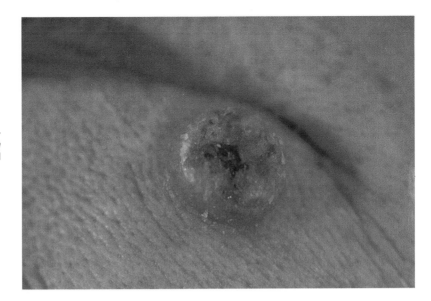

KERATOACANTHOMA. Female; *age* 58 years; *duration* 4 months; lower lip; confirmed by biopsy.

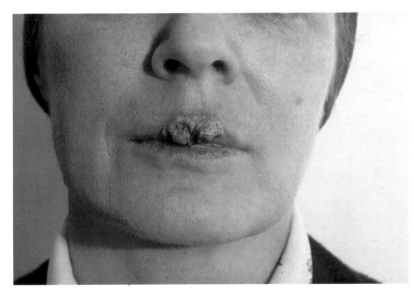

KERATOACANTHOMA. Female; *age* 49 years; *duration* 18 weeks; upper lip; confirmed by biopsy.

KERATOACANTHOMA (SPONTANEOUS REGRESSION). Female; *age* 49 years; *duration* 6 months; upper lip; confirmed by biopsy. (Same patient as in previous photograph.)

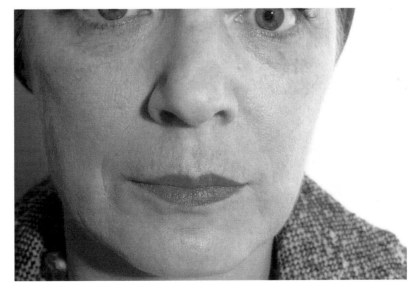

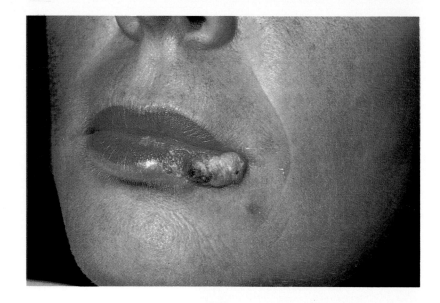

KERATOACANTHOMA. Female; lower lip; confirmed by biopsy.

KERATOACANTHOMA. Male; lower lip.

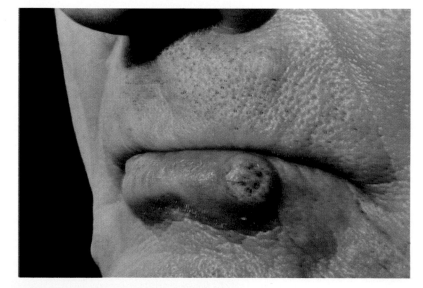

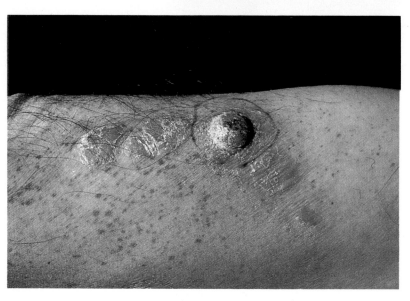

KERATOACANTHOMA, ARISING IN PSORIASIS. Male; forearm; confirmed by biopsy.

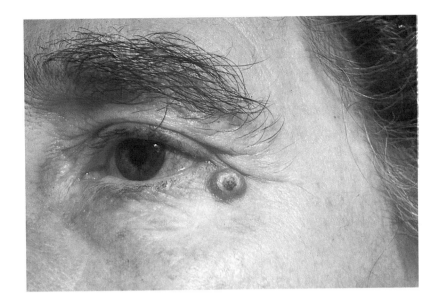

KERATOACANTHOMA ARISING IN RADIODERMATITIS. Female; lower eyelid; confirmed by biopsy.

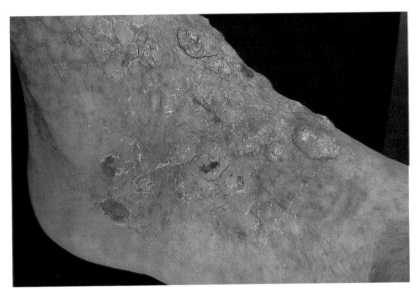

KERATOACANTHOMA (MULTIPLE). Female; foot.

KERATOACANTHOMA (MULTIPLE). Male; *age* 27 years; *duration* 17 years; ankles; confirmed by biopsy.

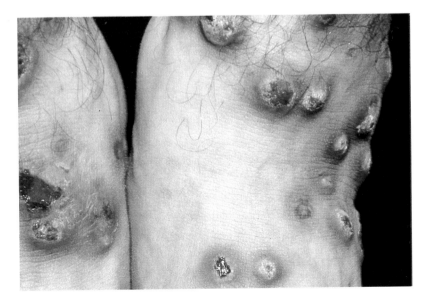

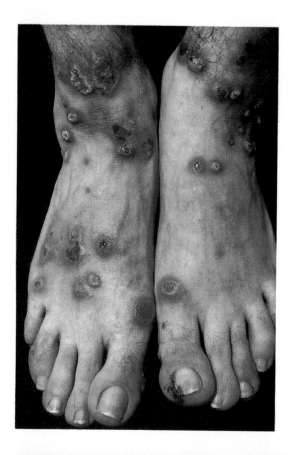

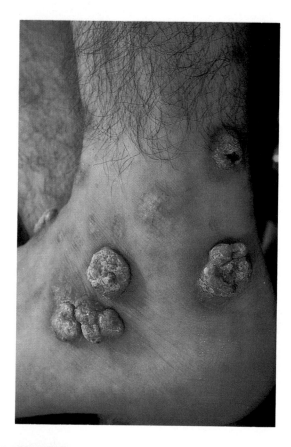

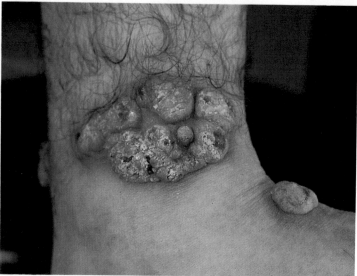

KERATOACANTHOMA (MULTIPLE). Male; *age* 27 years; *duration* 17 years; feet and ankles; confirmed by biopsy. (Same patient as in previous photograph.) (*top left*)

KERATOACANTHOMA (MULTIPLE). Male; *age* 27 years; *duration* 17 years; extremities; confirmed by biopsy. (Same patient as in previous photograph.) (*top right*)

KERATOACANTHOMA (MULTIPLE). Male; *age* 29 years; *duration* 19 years; ankle; confirmed by biopsy. (Same patient as in previous photograph.)

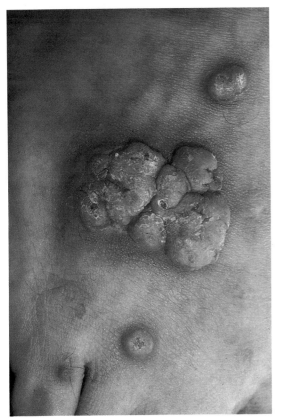

KERATOACANTHOMA (MULTIPLE). Male; dorsum of foot; confirmed by biopsy. (Same patient as in previous photograph.)

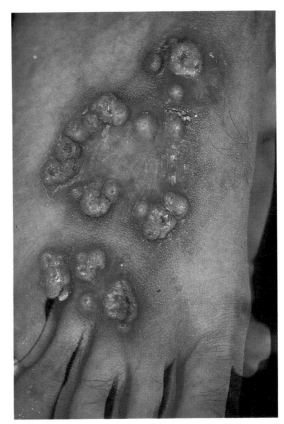

KERATOACANTHOMA (MULTIPLE). Male; *age 27* years; *duration* 17 years; extremities; confirmed by biopsy. (Same patient as in previous photographs.)

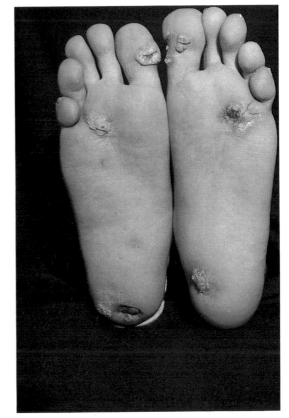

KERATOACANTHOMA (MULTIPLE). Male; soles; confirmed by biopsy. (Same patient as in previous photograph.)

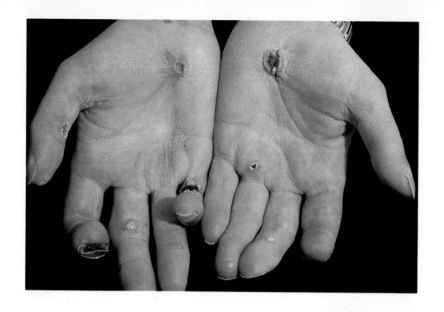

KERATOACANTHOMA (MULTIPLE). Male; palms and fingers; confirmed by biopsy. (Same patient as in previous photograph.)

KERATOACANTHOMA (MULTIPLE). Male; fingers and palms; confirmed by biopsy. (Same patient as in previous photograph.)

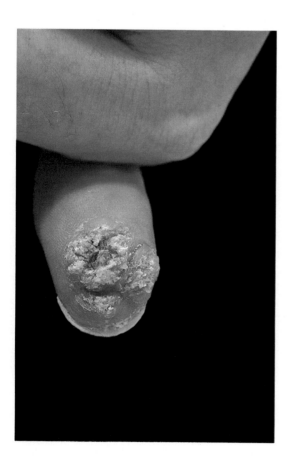

KERATOACANTHOMA (MULTIPLE). Male; *age* 29 years; *duration* 19 years; thumb; confirmed by biopsy. (Same patient as in previous photographs.)

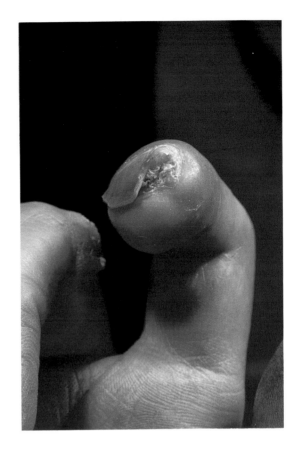

KERATOACANTHOMA (MUL-TIPLE). Male; *age* 24 years; *duration* 14 years; index finger; confirmed by biopsy. (Same patient as in previous photograph.)

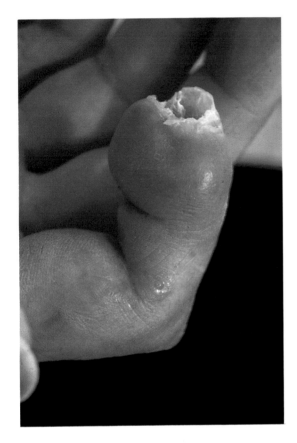

KERATOACANTHOMA (MUL-TIPLE). Male; index finger; confirmed by biopsy. (Same patient as in previous photograph.)

KERATOACANTHOMA (MUL-TIPLE) AT GRAFT DONOR SITE. Male; thigh; confirmed by biopsy. (Same patient as in previous photograph.)

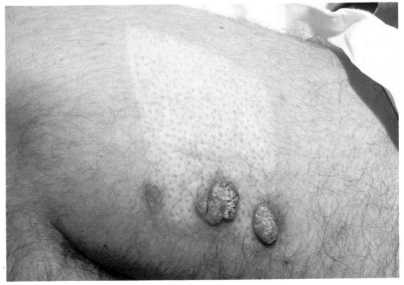

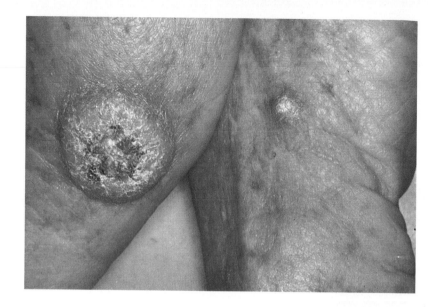

**KERATOACANTHOMA (GI-
ANT).** Male; wrist; confirmed
by biopsy.

**KERATOACANTHOMA (GI-
ANT).** Female; *age* 67 years;
duration 6 months; hand; confirmed by biopsy.

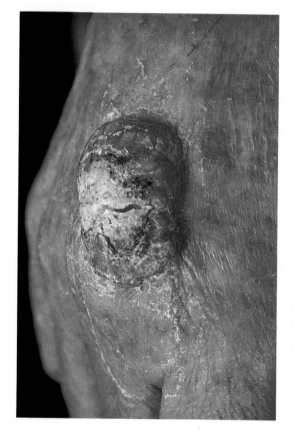

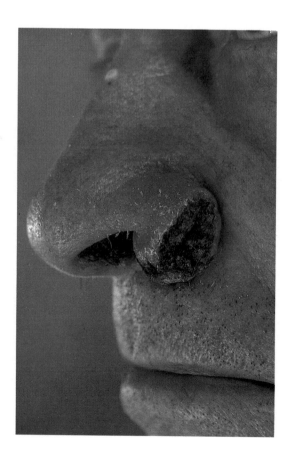

**KERATOACANTHOMA (GI-
ANT).** Male; *age* 78 years;
duration 3 months; ala nasi.

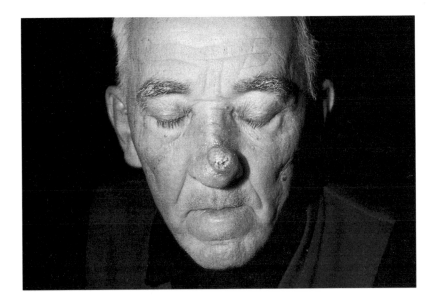

KERATOACANTHOMA (GI-ANT). Male; *duration* 2 months; nose; confirmed by biopsy.

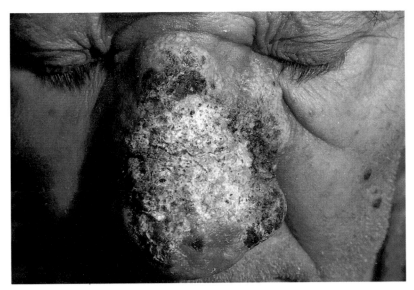

KERATOACANTHOMA (GI-ANT). Male; *age* 67 years; *duration* 4 months; nose; confirmed by biopsy. (Same patient as in previous photograph.)

KERATOACANTHOMA (GI-ANT). Male; *age* 67 years; *duration* 4 months; nose; confirmed by biopsy. (Same patient as in previous photograph.)

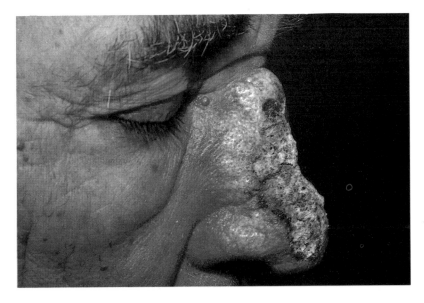

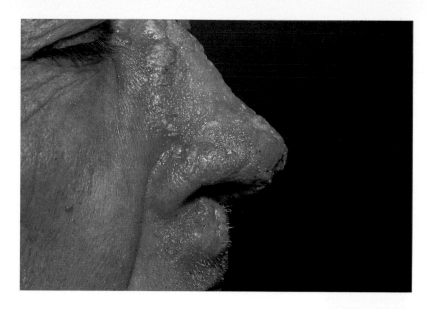

KERATOACANTHOMA (GIANT) (SPONTANEOUS INVOLUTION). Male; *age* 67 years; *duration* 6 months; nose; confirmed by biopsy. (Same patient as in previous photograph.)

KERATOACANTHOMA (GIANT) (FURTHER SPONTANEOUS INVOLUTION). Male; *age* 69 years; *duration* 3 years; nose; confirmed by biopsy. (Same patient as in previous photograph.)

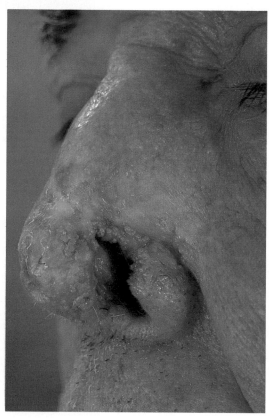

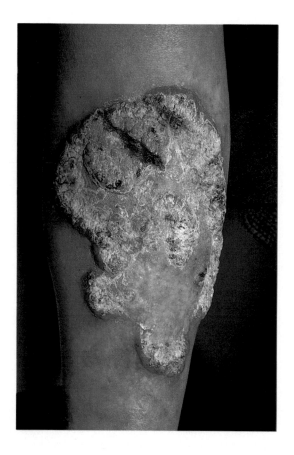

KERATOACANTHOMA (GIANT). Male; *age* 66 years; *duration* 2 years; leg; confirmed by biopsy.

KERATOACANTHOMA (GIANT). Male; leg; confirmed by biopsy.

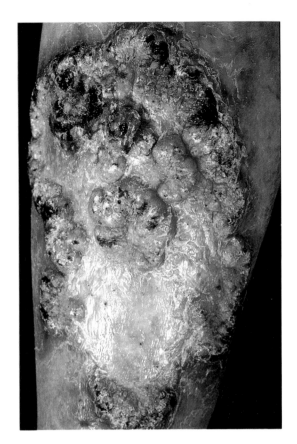

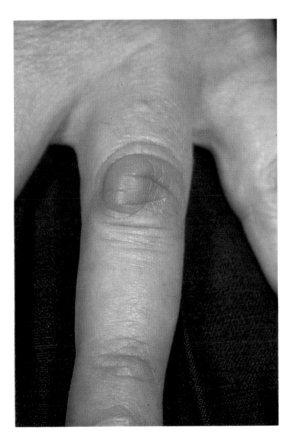

KNUCKLE PAD. Female; *age* 47 years; finger.

LEIOMYOMAS. Male; *age* 69 years; *duration* 25 years; face; confirmed by biopsy.

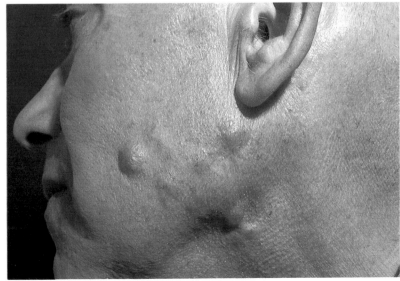

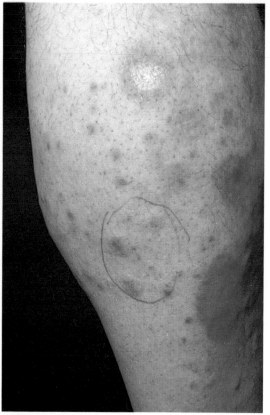

LEIOMYOMAS. Male; *age* 37 years; *duration* 12 years; leg; confirmed by biopsy.

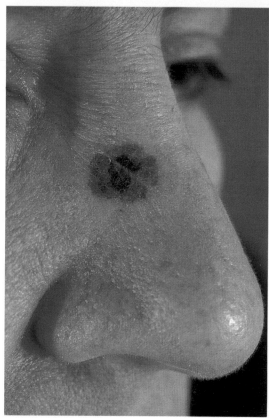

LENTIGO MALIGNA. Female; *age* 46 years; *duration* 6 years; nose; confirmed by biopsy.

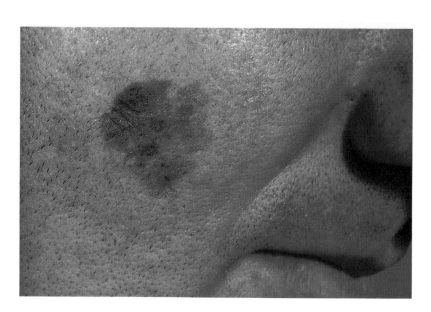

LENTIGO MALIGNA. Male; *age* 21 years; *duration* 3 years; cheek; confirmed by biopsy.

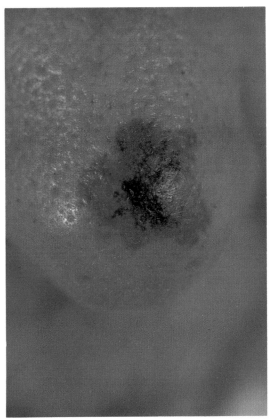

LENTIGO MALIGNA. Female; *age* 58 years; *duration* 2 years; nose; confirmed by biopsy.

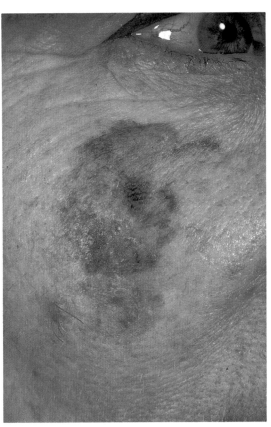

LENTIGO MALIGNA. Female; *age* 65 years; *duration* 2 years; cheek; confirmed by biopsy.

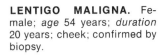

LENTIGO MALIGNA. Female; *age* 54 years; *duration* 20 years; cheek; confirmed by biopsy.

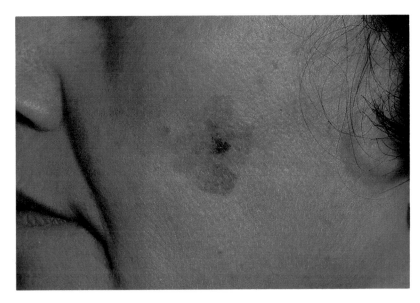

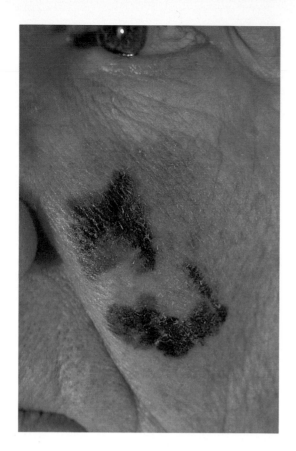

LENTIGO MALIGNA. Male; cheek; confirmed by biopsy.

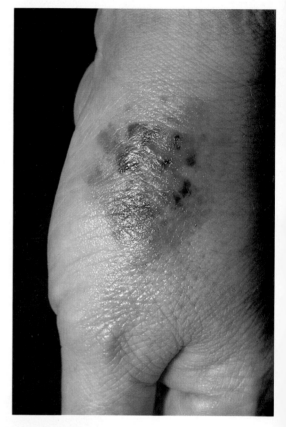

LENTIGO MALIGNA. Female; *age* 58 years; *duration* 10 years; hand; confirmed by biopsy.

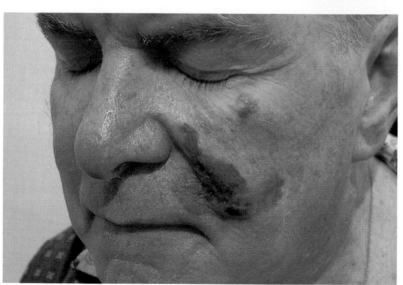

LENTIGO MALIGNA. Male; *age* 64 years; *duration* 10 years; cheek; confirmed by biopsy.

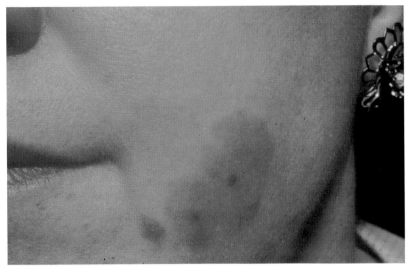

LENTIGO MALIGNA. Female; *age* 46 years; *duration* 5 years; cheek; confirmed by biopsy.

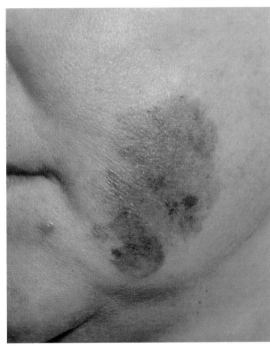

LENTIGO MALIGNA. Female; *age* 49 years; *duration* 8 years; cheek; confirmed by biopsy. (Same patient as in previous photograph.)

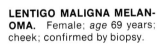

LENTIGO MALIGNA MELAN-OMA. Female; *age* 69 years; cheek; confirmed by biopsy.

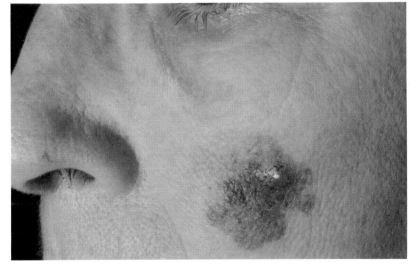

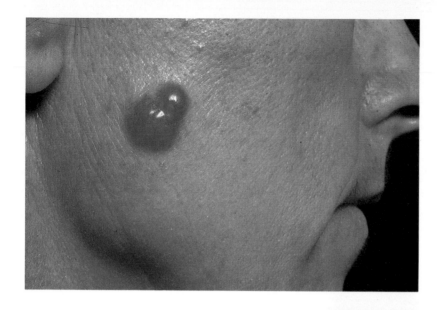

LEUKEMIA CUTIS. Female; *age* 48 years; *duration* 8 years; face; confirmed by biopsy.

LEUKEMIA CUTIS. Male; *age* 67 years; face; confirmed by biopsy.

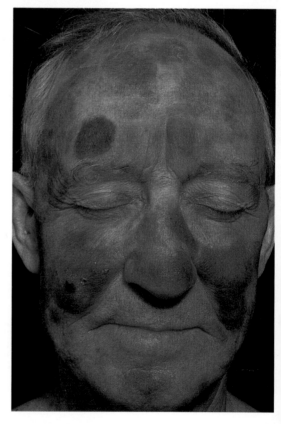

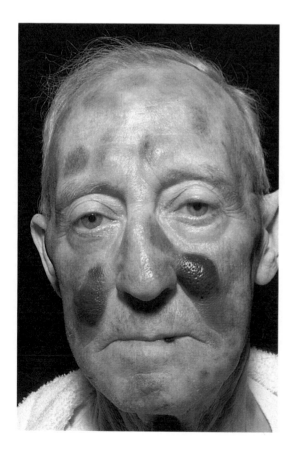

LEUKEMIA CUTIS. Male; *age* 68 years; face; confirmed by biopsy. (Same patient as in previous photograph, 3 months later.)

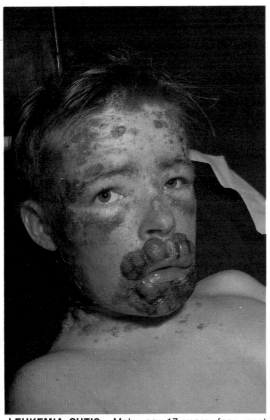

LEUKEMIA CUTIS. Male; *age* 17 years; face, neck.

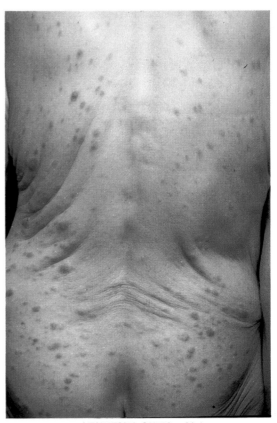

LEUKEMIA CUTIS. Male.

LEUKEMIA CUTIS. Male; *age* 77 years; *duration* 3 weeks; scalp; confirmed by biopsy.

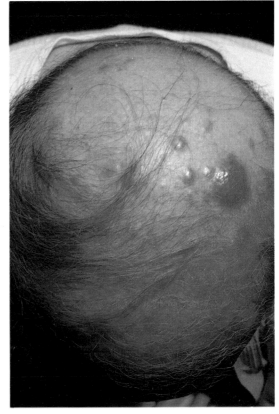

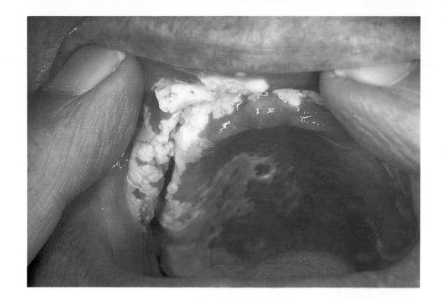

LEUKOPLAKIA. Male; *age* 58 years; *duration* 1 year; mouth; confirmed by biopsy.

LEUKOPLAKIA. Female; *age* adult; *duration* unknown; gingiva.

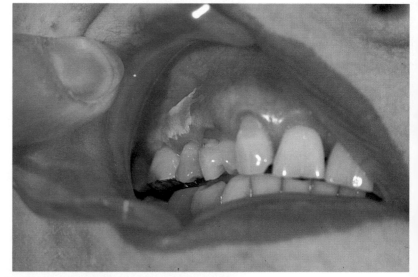

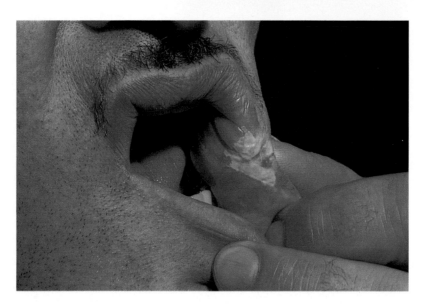

LEUKOPLAKIA. Male; *age* 46 years; *duration* 10 years; oral commissure; confirmed by biopsy.

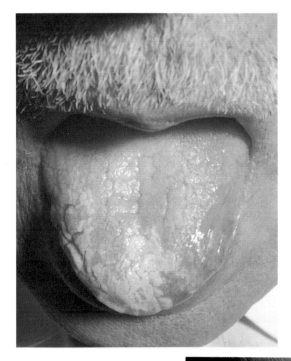

LEUKOPLAKIA. Male; *age* 72 years; *duration* 10 years; tongue; confirmed by biopsy.

LIPOMA. Male; *age* 70 years; *duration* 9 years; thigh.

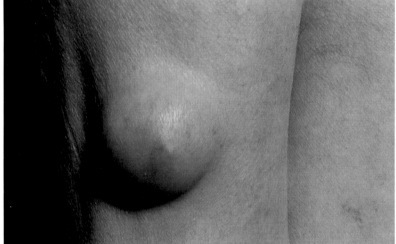

LIPOMA. Male; *age* 48 years; leg; confirmed by biopsy.

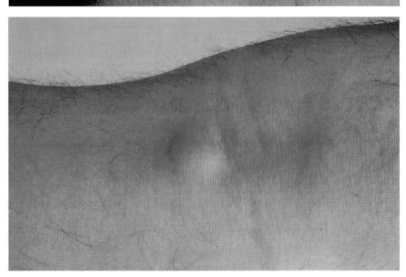

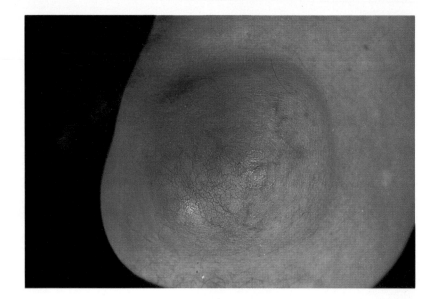

LIPOMA. Male; *age* 58 years; *duration* 40 years; knee.

LIPOMA. Male; *age* 46 years; *duration* 1 year; thigh; confirmed by biopsy.

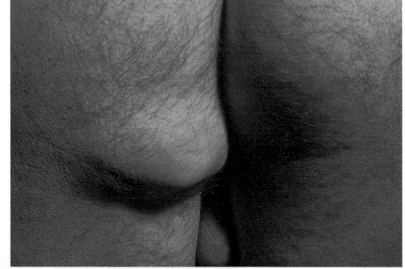

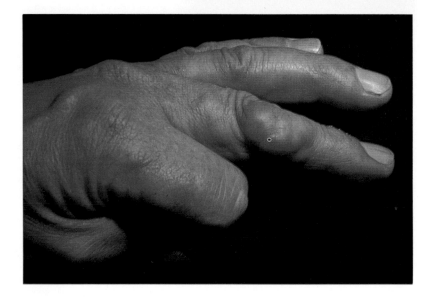

LIPOMA. Male; *age* 66 years; *duration* 39 years; middle finger; confirmed by biopsy.

LIPOMATOSIS. Male; neck.

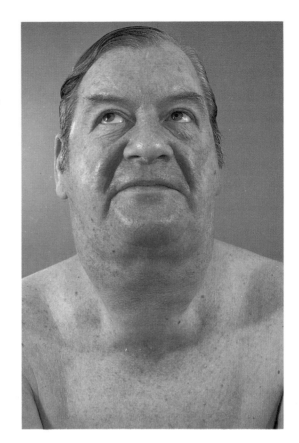

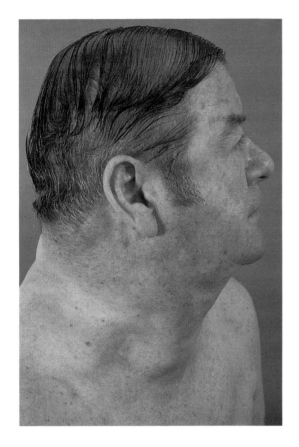

LIPOMATOSIS. Male; neck.
(Same patient as in previous
photograph.)

LIPOMATOSIS. Male; *age* 37
years; *duration* 5 years; lower
extremity; confirmed by biopsy.

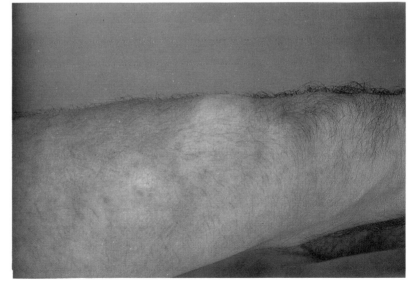

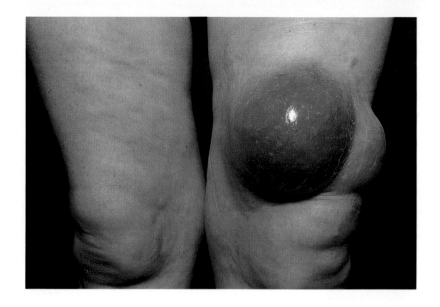

LIPOSARCOMA. Female; *age* 59 years; *duration* 5 years; thigh; confirmed by biopsy.

LYMPHANGIOMA. Female; *age* one-and-a-half years; *duration* since birth; thorax; confirmed by biopsy.

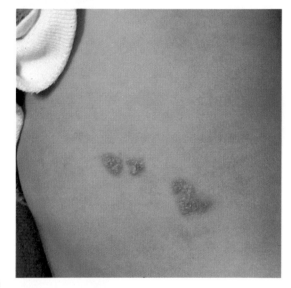

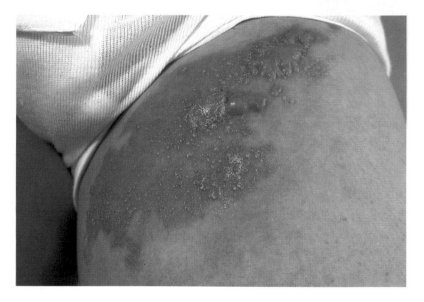

LYMPHANGIOMA. Male; *age* 9 years; *duration* 2 years; thigh; confirmed by biopsy.

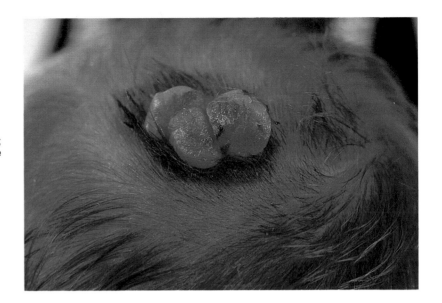

LYMPHANGIOMA. Female; *age* 5 days; *duration* since birth; scalp.

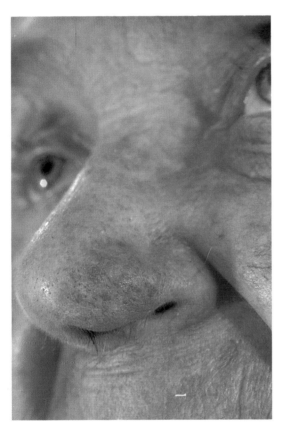

LYMPHANGIOMA. Female; *age* 71 years; *duration* 9 years; nose; confirmed by biopsy.

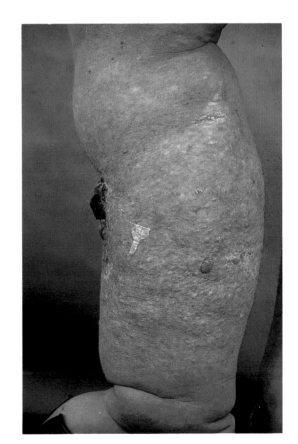

LYMPHANGIOSARCOMA. Female; *age* 52 years; leg; confirmed by biopsy. (Twenty years after groin dissection for malignant melanoma.)

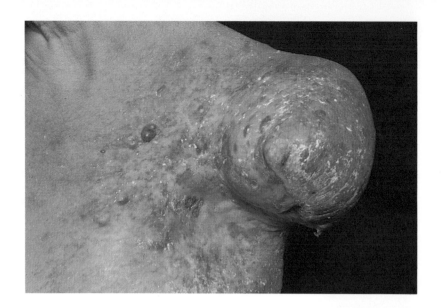

LYMPHANGIOSARCOMA (AFTER MASTECTOMY). Female; upper extremity and thorax.

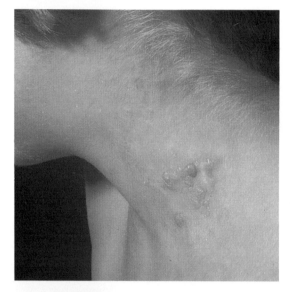

LYMPH-HEMANGIOMA. Female; *age* 4 years; *duration* since birth; neck; confirmed by biopsy.

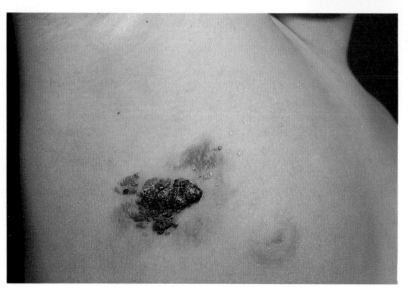

LYMPH - HEMANGIOMA. Male; *age* 8 years; *duration* since birth; chest; confirmed by biopsy.

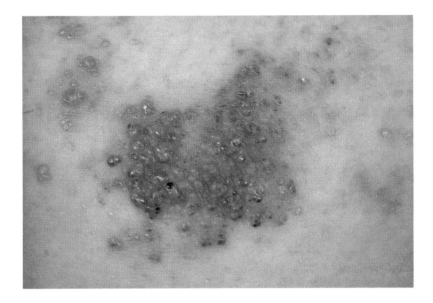

LYMPH - HEMANGIOMA.
Male; *age* 15 years; *duration*
since birth; thigh; confirmed
by biopsy.

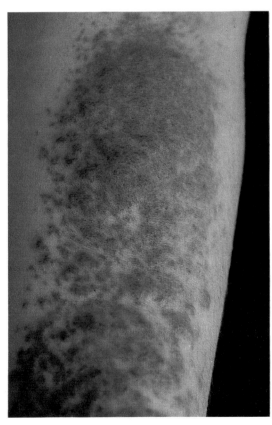

LYMPH - HEMANGIOMA.
Age 23 years; *duration* since
birth; upper extremity.

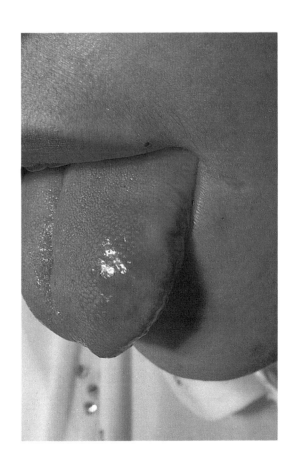

LYMPH - HEMANGIOMA.
Female; tongue.

LYMPHOCYTIC INFILTRA-TIONS OF THE SKIN. Male; *age* 39 years; *duration* 6 weeks; face; confirmed by biopsy.

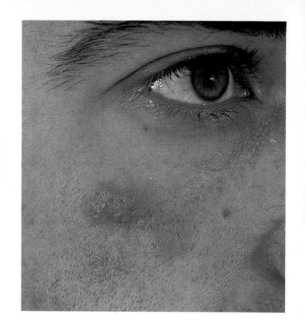

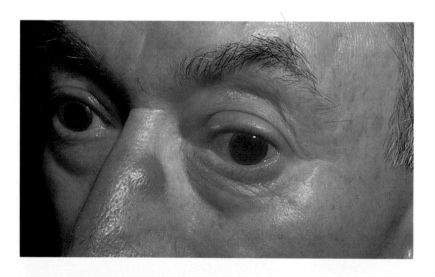

LYMPHOCYTOMA CUTIS. Male; nose.

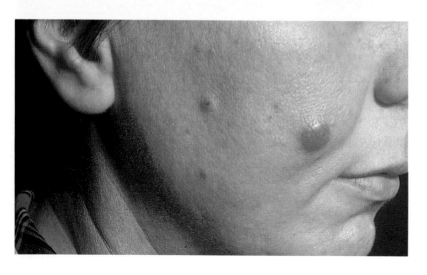

LYMPHOCYTOMA CUTIS. Female; *age* 45 years; *duration* 1 month; face.

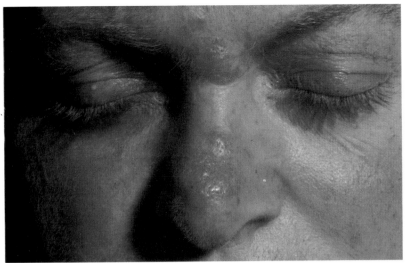

LYMPHOCYTOMA CUTIS.
Female; *age* 40 years; *duration* 1 month; forehead; confirmed by biopsy.

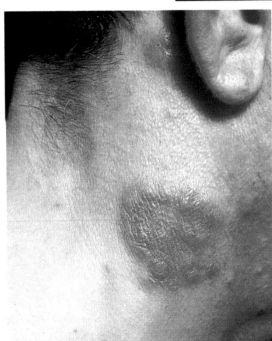

LYMPHOCYTOMA CUTIS.
Male; *age* 47 years; *duration* 4 years; neck; confirmed by biopsy.

LYMPHOCYTOMA CUTIS.
Male; *age* 47 years; *duration* 4 years; neck; confirmed by biopsy. (Same patient as in previous photograph.)

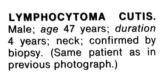
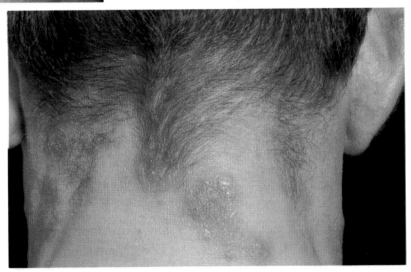

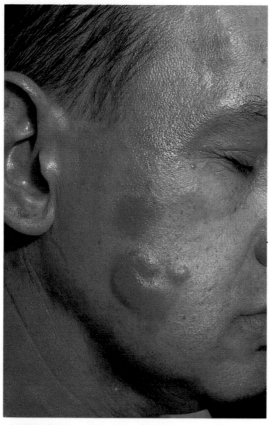

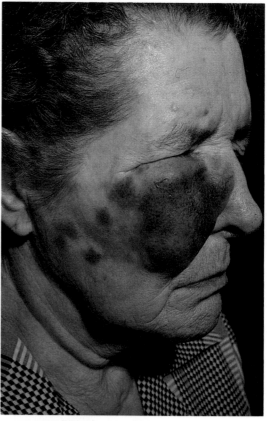

LYMPHOMA. Male; *age* 48 years; *duration* 8 years; cheek and neck; confirmed by biopsy.

LYMPHOMA. Female; *age* 67 years; face.

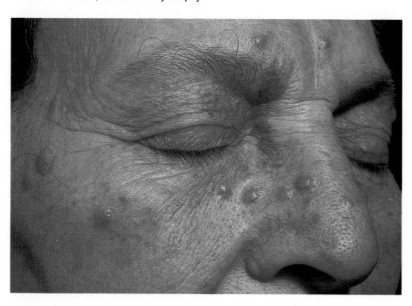

LYMPHOMA. female; *age* 67 years; *duration* 6 months; face; confirmed by biopsy.

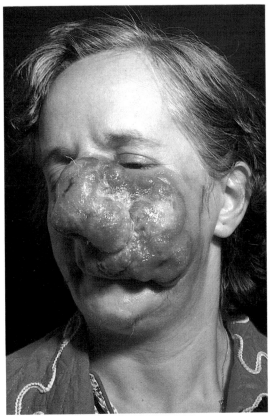

LYMPHOMA. Female; *age* 42 years; *duration* 1 year; face; confirmed by biopsy.

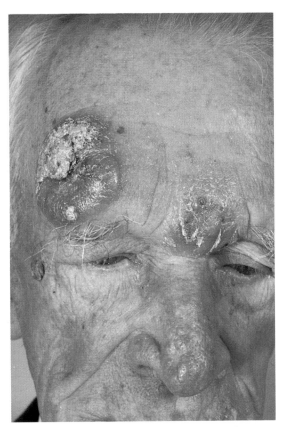

LYMPHOMA. Male; *age* 76 years; *duration* 1½ years; forehead; confirmed by biopsy.

LYMPHOMA. Male; *age* 52 years; head and trunk; confirmed by biopsy.

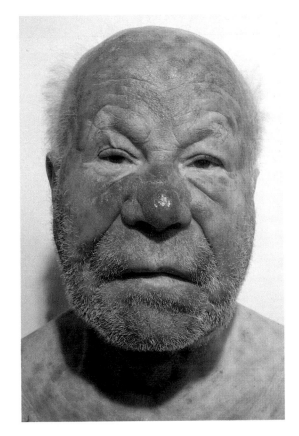

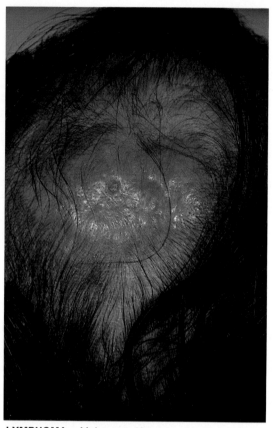

LYMPHOMA. Male; *age* 46 years; *duration* 7 years; scalp; confirmed by biopsy.

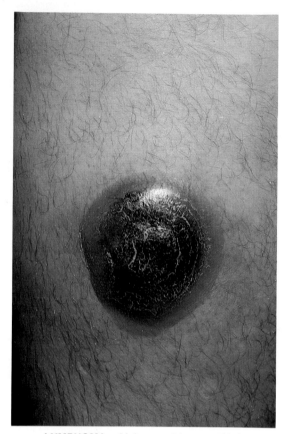

LYMPHOMA. Male; *age* 54 years; thigh.

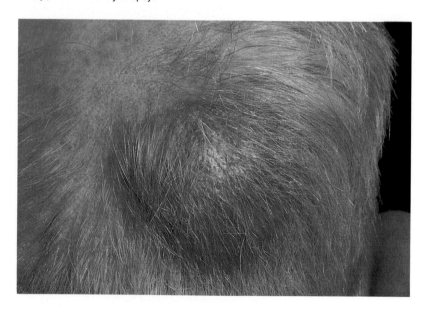

LYMPHOMA. Male; *age* 76 years; *duration* 2 months; occipital region; confirmed by biopsy.

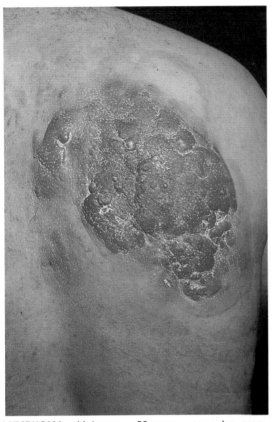

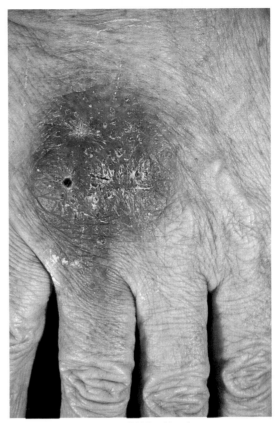

LYMPHOMA. Male; *age* 52 years; scapular area; confirmed by biopsy.

LYMPHOMA. Hand.

LYMPHOMA. Male; *age* 54 years; *duration* 15 months; arm; confirmed by biopsy.

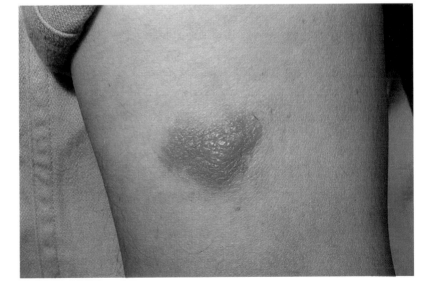

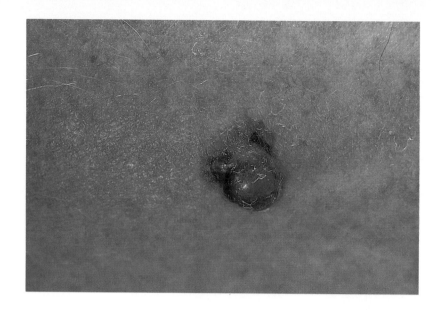

MALIGNANT MELANOMA (SUPERFICIAL SPREADING). Male; *age* 70 years; *duration* 20 years; arm; confirmed by biopsy.

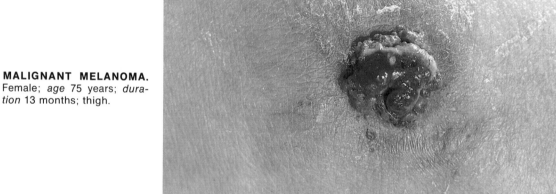

MALIGNANT MELANOMA. Female; *age* 75 years; *duration* 13 months; thigh.

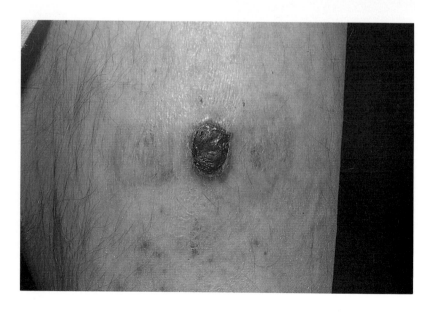

MALIGNANT MELANOMA, NODULAR. Male; *age* 69 years; *duration* 7 months; thigh; confirmed by biopsy.

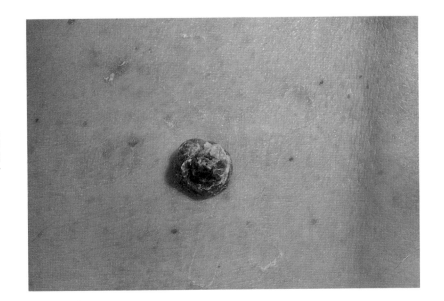

MALIGNANT MELANOMA. (NODULAR). Male; *age* 59 years; *duration* since birth; mid-back; confirmed by biopsy.

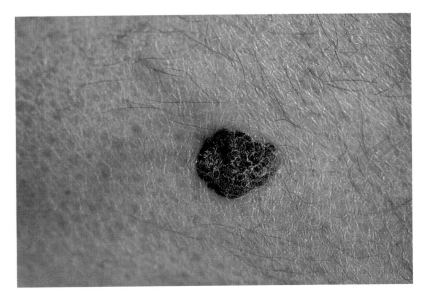

MALIGNANT MELANOMA. (TYPE UNCLASSIFIED). Male; *age* 44 years; *duration* since birth; calf; confirmed by biopsy.

MALIGNANT MELANOMA. (SUPERFICIAL SPREADING). Female; *age* 44 years; *duration* 6 months; anterior aspect; confirmed by biopsy.

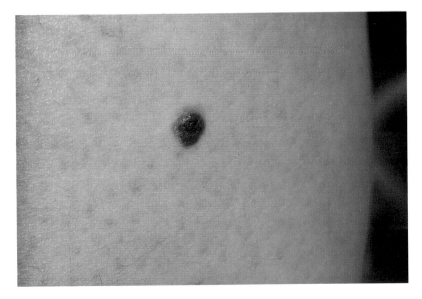

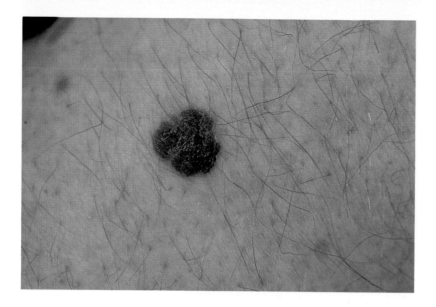

**MALIGNANT MELANOMA.
(SUPERFICIAL SPREADING).**
Female; *age* 74 years; *duration* 13 months; leg; confirmed by biopsy.

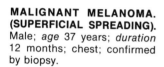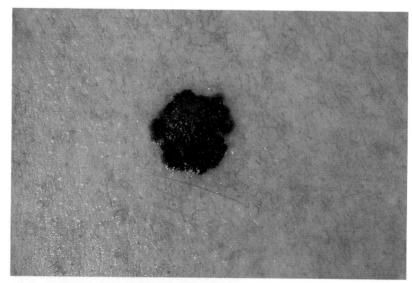

**MALIGNANT MELANOMA.
(SUPERFICIAL SPREADING).**
Male; *age* 37 years; *duration* 12 months; chest; confirmed by biopsy.

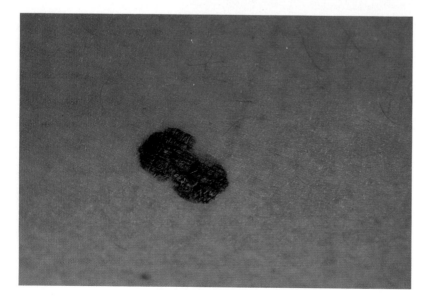

**MALIGNANT MELANOMA.
(SUPERFICIAL SPREADING).**
Confirmed by biopsy.

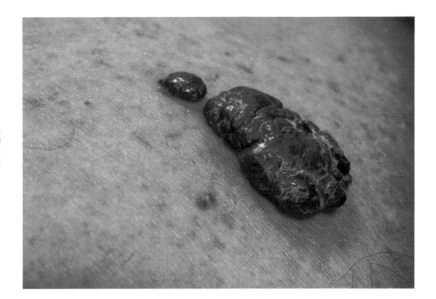

MALIGNANT MELANOMA. (NODULAR). Male; *age* 69 years; *duration* 13 months; shoulder; confirmed by biopsy.

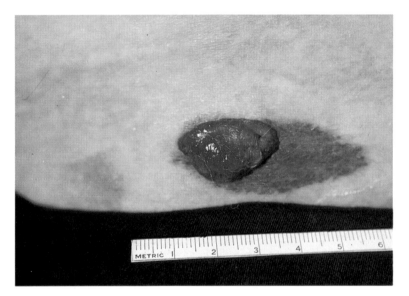
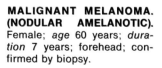

MALIGNANT MELANOMA, ARISING IN A CONGENITAL NEVOCYTIC NEVUS. Female; *age* 37 years; *duration* nevus present since birth; hip; confirmed by biopsy.

MALIGNANT MELANOMA. (NODULAR AMELANOTIC). Female; *age* 60 years; *duration* 7 years; forehead; confirmed by biopsy.

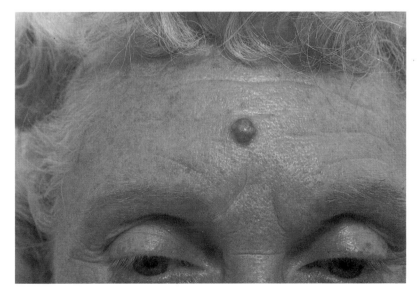

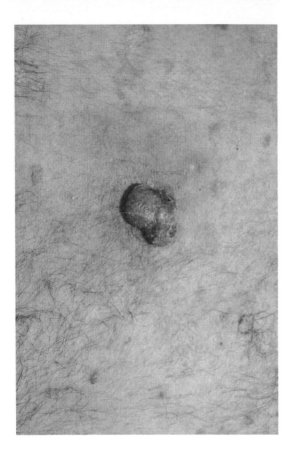

**MALIGNANT MELANOMA.
(AMELANOTIC).** Confirmed
by biopsy.

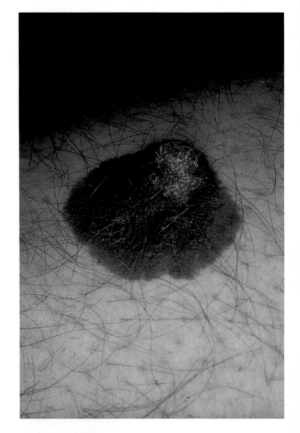

**MALIGNANT MELANOMA.
(TYPE UNCLASSIFIED).**
Male; *age* 41 years; *duration*
6 months; calf; confirmed by
biopsy.

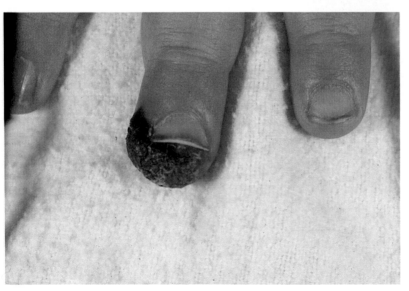

**MALIGNANT MELANOMA.
(CONGENITAL).** Male; *age*
11 months; *duration* since
birth; finger; confirmed by
biopsy. (This melanoma metastasized to the axillary lymph
nodes.)

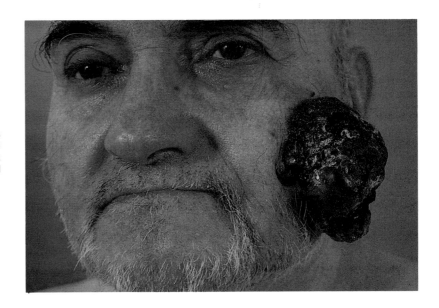

MALIGNANT MELANOMA (NODULAR). Male; *age* 66 years; *duration* one-and-a half years; cheek; confirmed by biopsy.

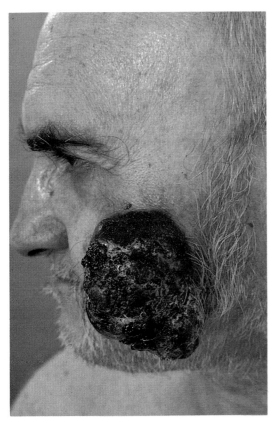

MALIGNANT MELANOMA (NODULAR). Male; *age* 66 years; *duration* one-and-a half years; cheek; confirmed by biopsy. (Same patient as in previous photograph.)

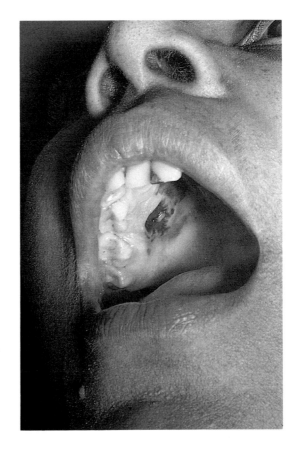

MALIGNANT MELANOMA. Female; *age* 42 years; palate.

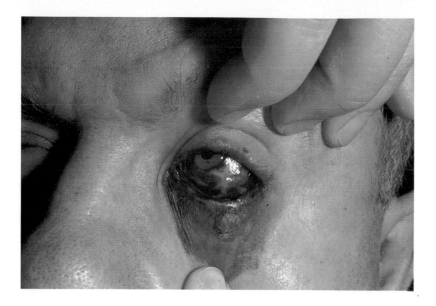

MALIGNANT MELANOMA.
Male; eye; confirmed by biopsy.

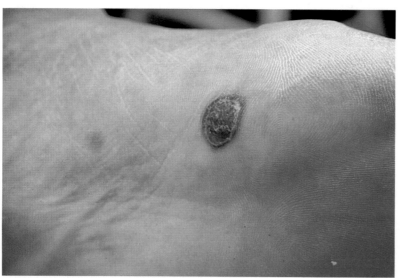

**MALIGNANT MELANOMA
(ACRAL LENTIGINOUS).** Female; *age* 73 years; *duration*
6 years; foot; confirmed by
biopsy.

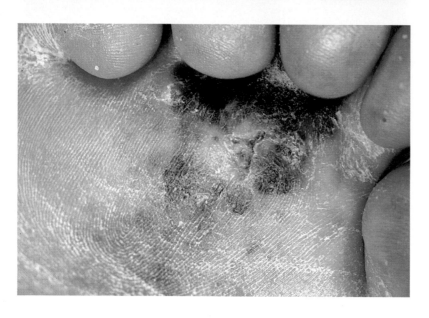

**MALIGNANT MELANOMA
(ACRAL LENTIGINOUS).**
Male; *age* 79 years; *duration*
6 months; sole.

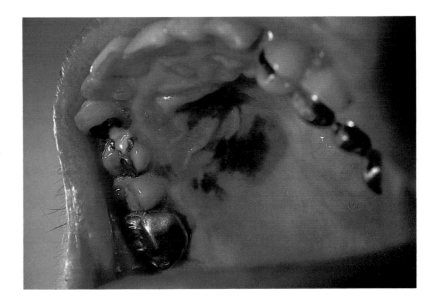

MALIGNANT MELANOMA.
Palate.

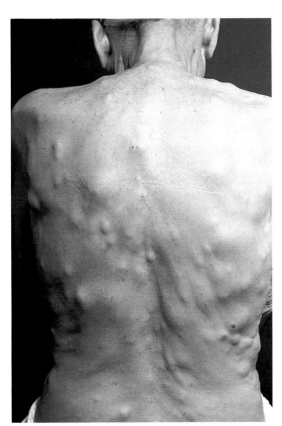

MALIGNANT MELANOMA (METASTATIC). Male; *age* 65 years; back; confirmed by biopsy.

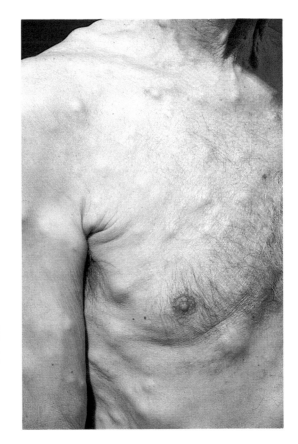

MALIGNANT MELANOMA.
Male; *age* 65 years; chest and arm; confirmed by biopsy. (Same patient as in previous photograph.)

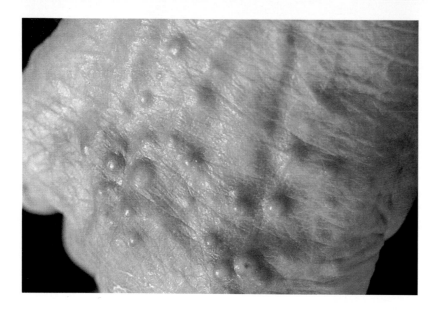

MALIGNANT MELANOMA (METASTATIC). Female; hand.

MALIGNANT MELANOMA (METASTATIC). Male; hip; confirmed by biopsy.

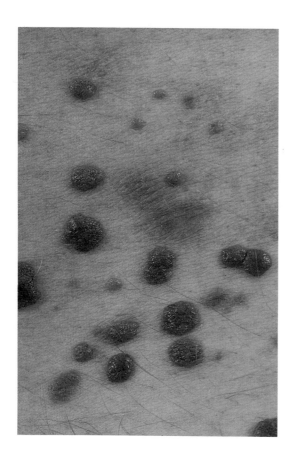

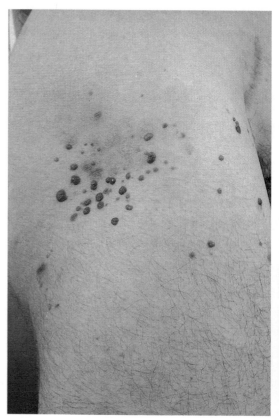

MALIGNANT MELANOMA (METASTATIC). Male; hip; confirmed by biopsy. (Same patient as in previous photograph.)

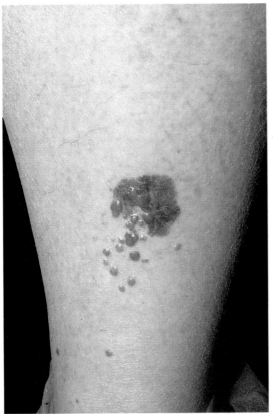

MALIGNANT MELANOMA (SATELLITOSIS). Female; *age* 45 years; *duration* 10 years; leg; confirmed by biopsy.

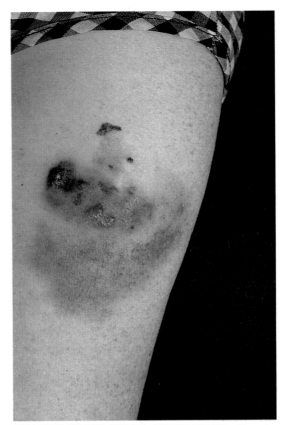

MALIGNANT MELANOMA (METASTATIC). Female; *age* 76 years; *duration* 20 years; arm; confirmed by biopsy.

MALIGNANT MELANOMA (METASTATIC). Toe and leg.

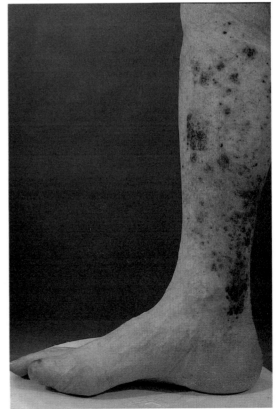

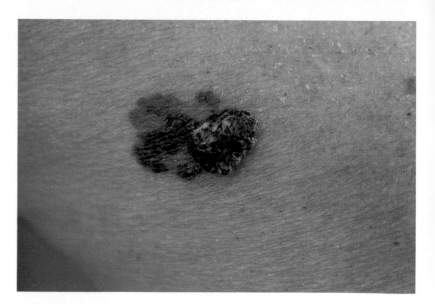

MALIGNANT MELANOMA (SUPERFICIAL SPREADING). Male; *age* unknown; sole.

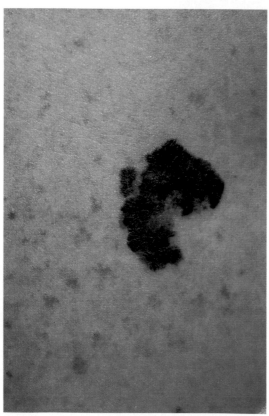

MALIGNANT MELANOMA (SUPERFICIAL SPREADING). Female; *age* 35 years; *duration* 19 years; anterior chest wall; confirmed by biopsy.

MALIGNANT MELANOMA (ACRAL-LENTIGINOUS). Female; *age* 58 years; *duration* 20 years; arm; confirmed by biopsy.

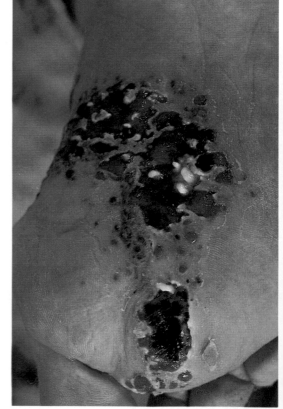

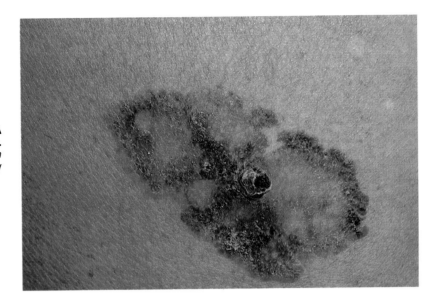

MALIGNANT MELANOMA (SUPERFICIAL SPREADING). Male; *age* 64 years; *duration* 10 years; back; confirmed by biopsy.

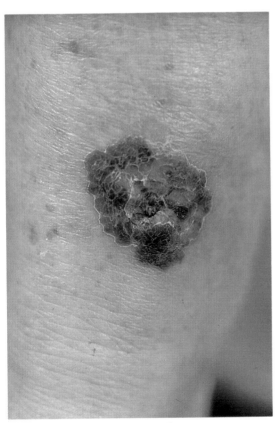

MALIGNANT MELANOMA. Female; *age* 70 years; *duration* 1 year; calf; confirmed by biopsy.

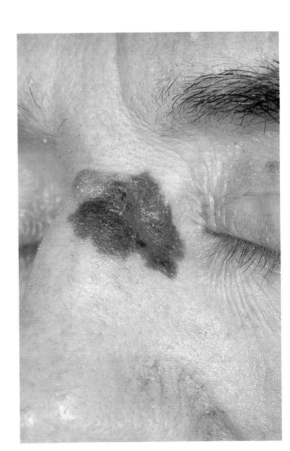

MALIGNANT MELANOMA (SUPERFICIAL SPREADING). Male; *age* 70 years; *duration* 20 years; nose; confirmed by biopsy.

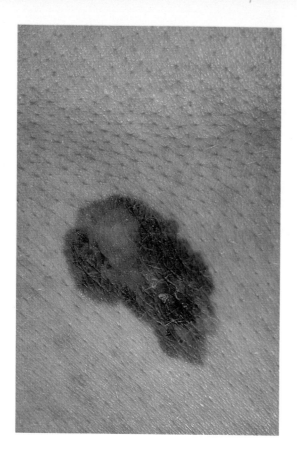

**MALIGNANT MELANOMA
(SUPERFICIAL SPREADING).**
Female; *age* 48 years; *duration* unknown; back; confirmed by biopsy.

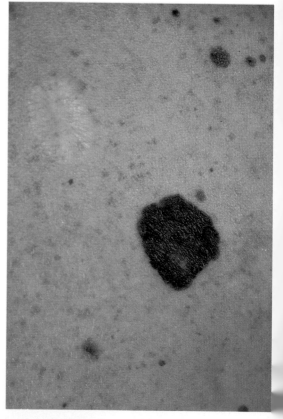

**MALIGNANT MELANOMA
(SUPERFICIAL SPREADING).**
Female; *age* 32 years; *duration* unknown; back; confirmed by biopsy.

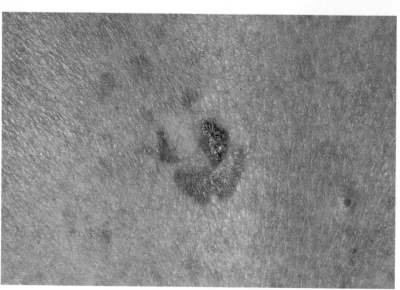

**MALIGNANT MELANOMA
(SUPERFICIAL SPREADING).**
Male; *age* 59 years; *duration* 13 months; back; confirmed by biopsy.

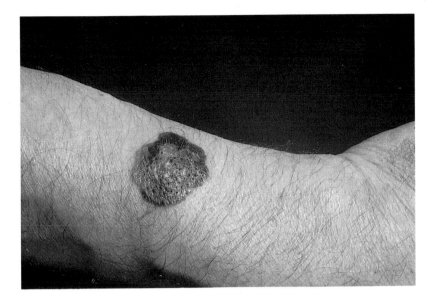

MALIGNANT MELANOMA (SUPERFICIAL SPREADING).
Male; *age* 69 years; wrist; confirmed by biopsy.

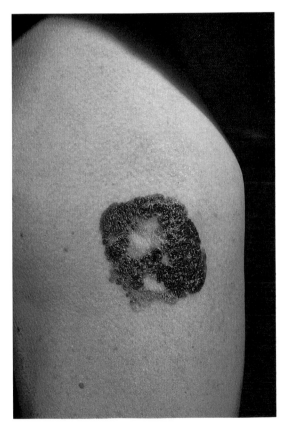

MALIGNANT MELANOMA (SUPERFICIAL SPREADING).
Female; *age* 67 years; *duration* 12 years; arm; confirmed by biopsy.

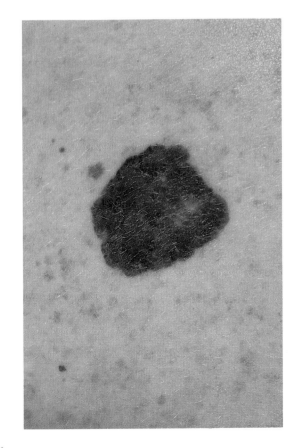

MALIGNANT MELANOMA (SUPERFICIAL SPREADING).
Female; *age* 61 years; *duration* 7 months; confirmed by biopsy.

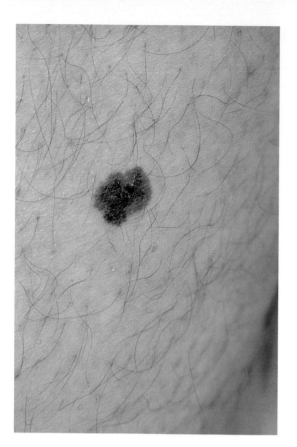

MALIGNANT MELANOMA (SUPERFICIAL SPREADING).
Male; *age* 51 years; *duration* 9 years; thigh; confirmed by biopsy.

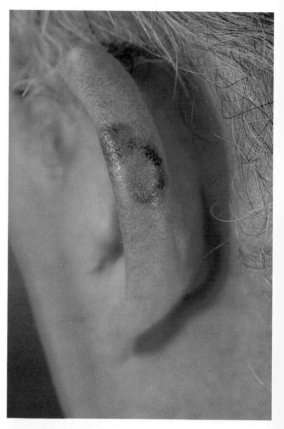

MALIGNANT MELANOMA.
Male; *age* 60 years; *duration* 5 years; rim of ear; confirmed by biopsy.

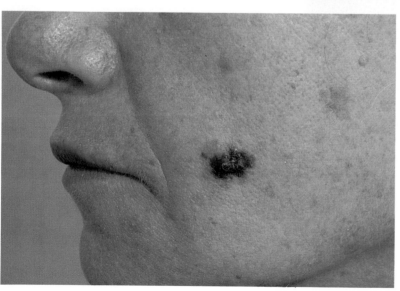

MALIGNANT MELANOMA (SUPERFICIAL SPREADING).
Female; *age* 61 years; *duration* 7 years; cheek; confirmed by biopsy.

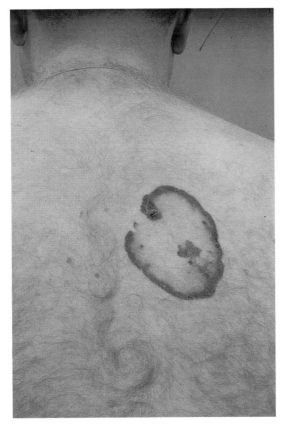

**MALIGNANT MELANOMA (SUPERFICIAL SPREAD-
ING).** Male; *duration* 15 years; trunk.

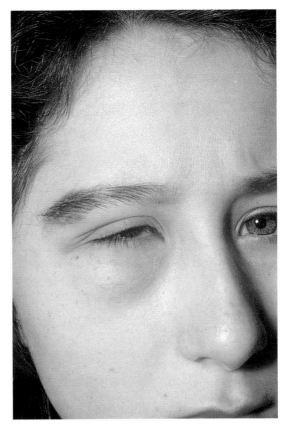

MELANOMA (MALIGNANT BLUE NEVUS). Female;
age 14 years; *duration* since birth; face; confirmed by
biopsy.

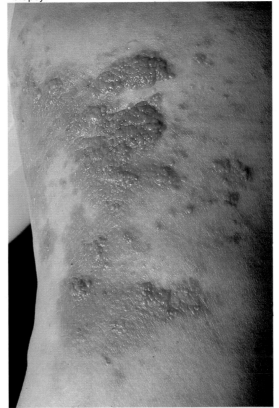

METASTATIC CARCINOMA (VULVAR). Female; *age*
61 years; arm; confirmed by biopsy.

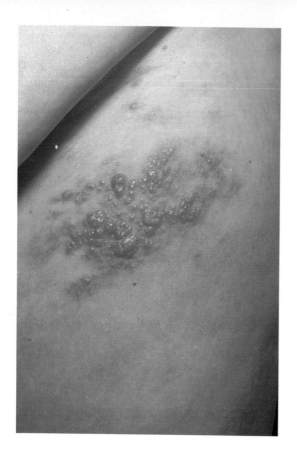

METASTATIC CARCINOMA (UNKNOWN PRIMARY). Female; *age* 73 years; *duration* 5–7 months; thigh; confirmed by biopsy.

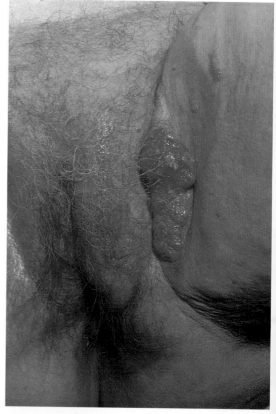

METASTATIC CARCINOMA (UNKNOWN PRIMARY). Female; *age* 73 years; *duration* 6 months; groin; confirmed by biopsy.

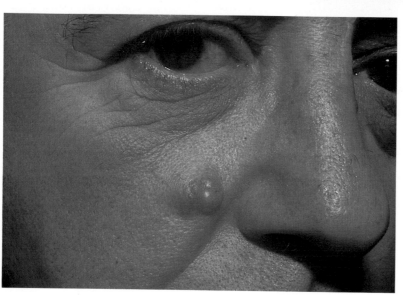

METASTATIC CARCINOMA (ANAPLASTIC; UNKNOWN PRIMARY). Male; *age* 52 years; *duration* 1 year; cheek; confirmed by biopsy.

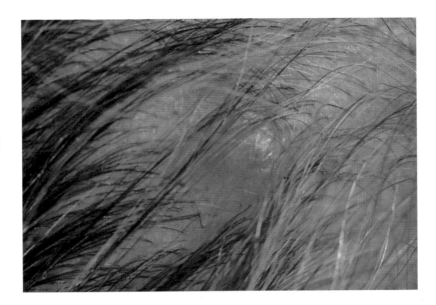

METASTATIC CARCINOMA (BREAST). Female; *age* 56 years; *duration* 10 months; scalp; confirmed by biopsy.

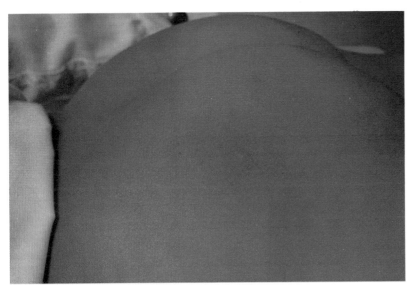

MONGOLIAN SPOT. Male; *age* 2 years; *duration* since birth; buttock.

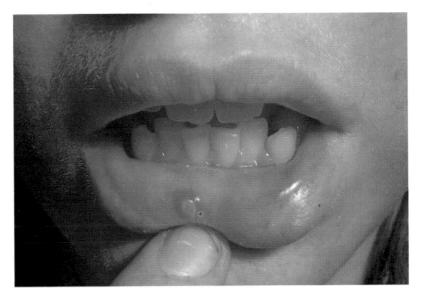

MUCOUS GLAND CYST. Female; *age* 19 years; *duration* 1 year; lower lip.

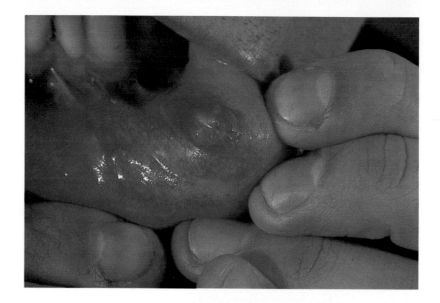

MUCOUS GLAND CYST.
Male; *age* 26 years; *duration* 4 months; buccal mucosa; confirmed by biopsy.

MUCOUS GLAND CYST.
Male; *age* 37 years; *duration* 5 weeks; lip.

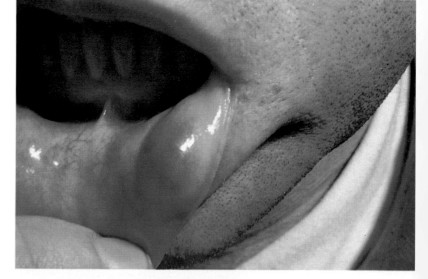

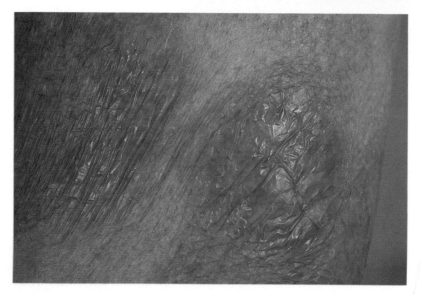

MYCOSIS FUNGOIDES. Female; *age* 64 years; *duration* 5 years; trunk; confirmed by biopsy.

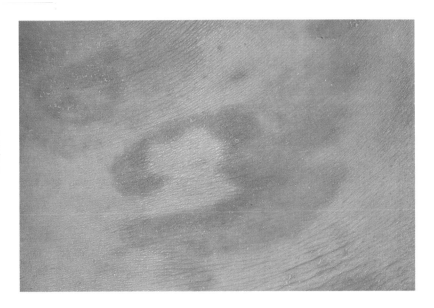

MYCOSIS FUNGOIDES. Female; *age* 64 years; *duration* 5 years; trunk; confirmed by biopsy. (Same patient as in previous photograph.)

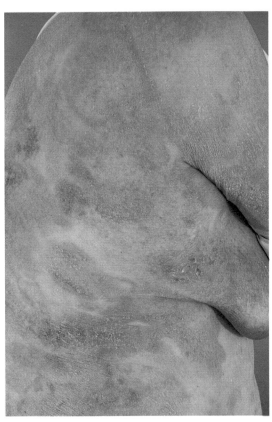

MYCOSIS FUNGOIDES. Female; *age* 64 years; *duration* 5 years; trunk and arm; confirmed by biopsy. (Same patient as in previous photograph.)

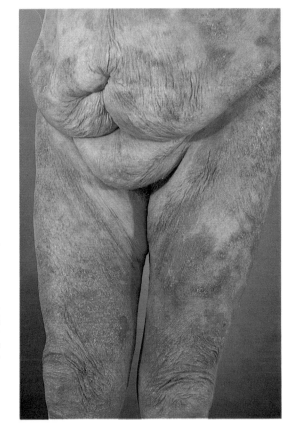

MYCOSIS FUNGOIDES. Female; *age* 64 years; *duration* 5 years; abdomen and thighs; confirmed by biopsy. (Same patient as in previous photograph.)

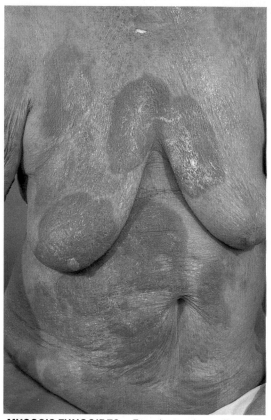

MYCOSIS FUNGOIDES. Female; trunk; confirmed by biopsy.

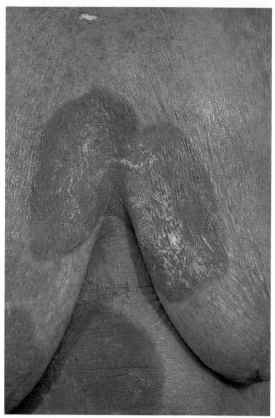

MYCOSIS FUNGOIDES. Female; chest; confirmed by biopsy. (Same patient as in previous photograph.)

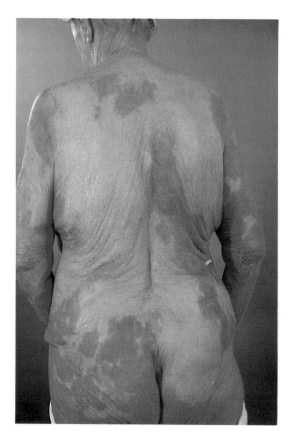

MYCOSIS FUNGOIDES. Female; trunk and upper extremities; confirmed by biopsy. (Same patient as in previous photograph.)

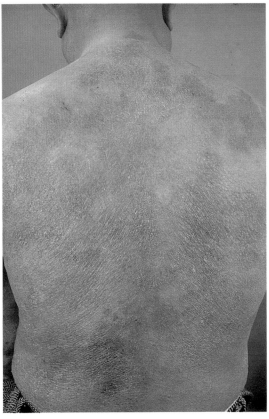

MYCOSIS FUNGOIDES. Male; *age* 57 years; back; confirmed by biopsy.

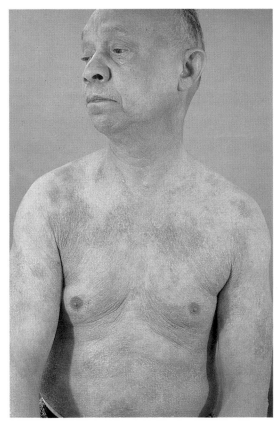

MYCOSIS FUNGOIDES. Male; *age* 57 years; face, chest and arms; confirmed by biopsy. (Same patient as in previous photograph.)

MYCOSIS FUNGOIDES. Male; *age* 57 years; *duration* 3 months; total body; confirmed by biopsy. (Same patient as in previous photograph.)

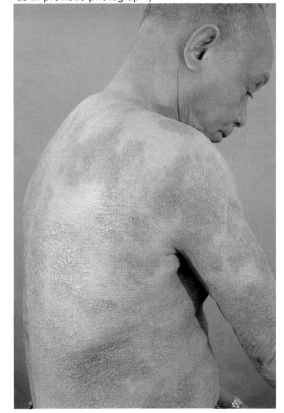

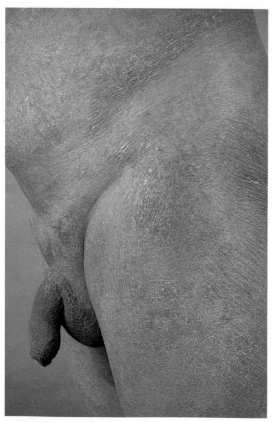

MYCOSIS FUNGOIDES. Male; *age* 57 years; abdomen and thigh; confirmed by biopsy.

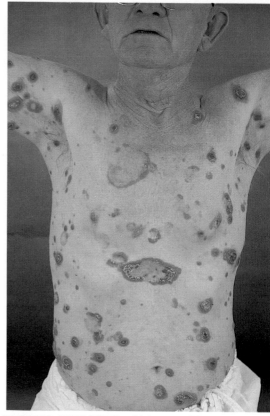

MYCOSIS FUNGOIDES. Male; *age* 75 years; trunk and arms; confirmed by biopsy.

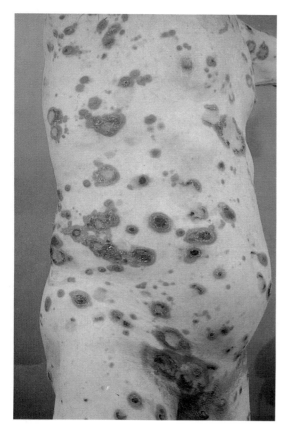

MYCOSIS FUNGOIDES. Male; *age* 75 years; trunk; confirmed by biopsy. (Same patient as in previous photograph.)

MYCOSIS FUNGOIDES.
Male; face; confirmed by biopsy.

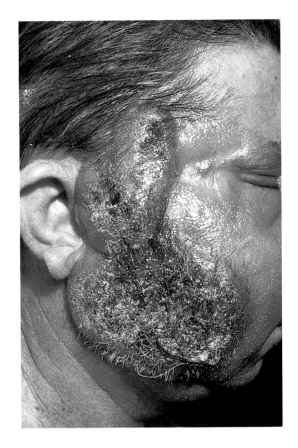

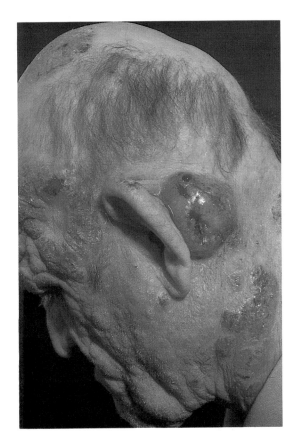

MYCOSIS FUNGOIDES.
Male; *age* 50 years; head and
neck; confirmed by biopsy.

MYCOSIS FUNGOIDES. Female; *age* 34 years; *duration*
7 years; shoulder; confirmed
by biopsy.

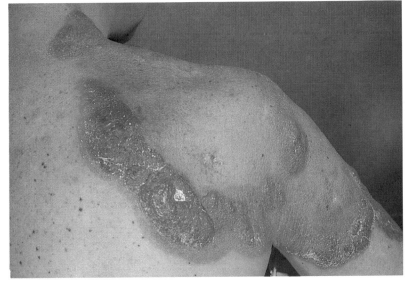

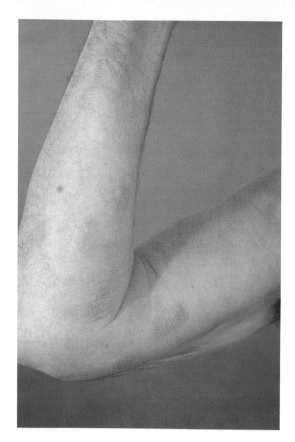

MYCOSIS FUNGOIDES.
Male; *age* 66 years; *duration* 5
years; upper extremity.

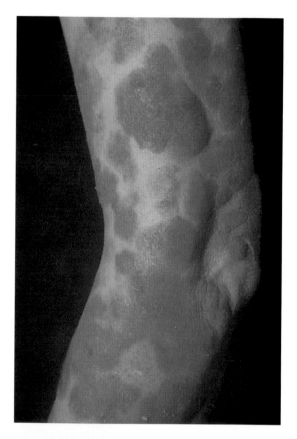

MYCOSIS FUNGOIDES. Female; *age* 44 years; upper extremity; confirmed by biopsy.

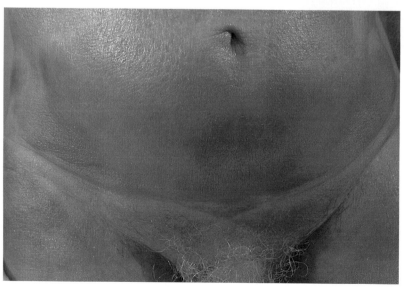

MYCOSIS FUNGOIDES.
Male; *age* 78 years; *duration*
40 years; abdomen; confirmed
by biopsy.

MYCOSIS FUNGOIDES.
Male; trunk and thigh.

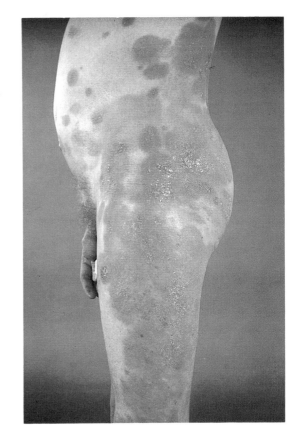

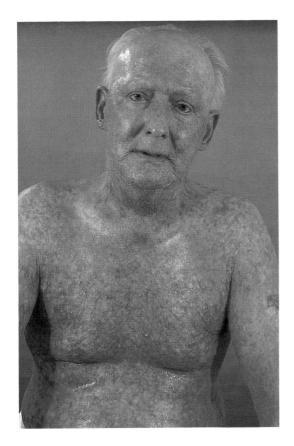

MYCOSIS FUNGOIDES.
Male; *age* 66 years; *duration*
5 years; head, neck and trunk;
confirmed by biopsy.

MYCOSIS FUNGOIDES.
Male; *age* 66 years; *duration* 5
years; chest and abdomen;
confirmed by biopsy. (Same
patient as in previous photograph.)

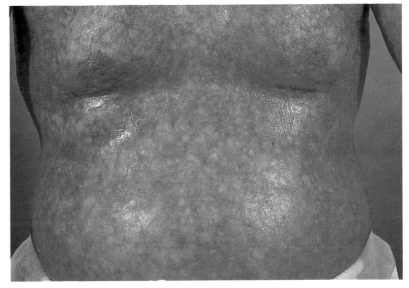

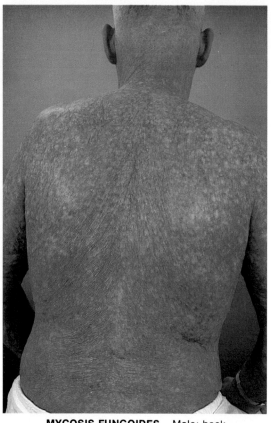

MYCOSIS FUNGOIDES.   Male; back.

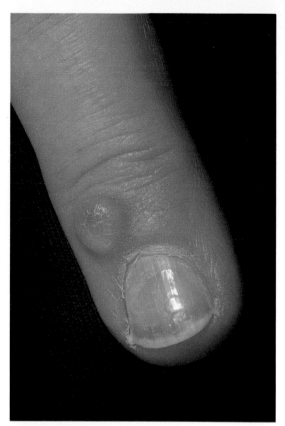

MYXOID DEGENERATION CYST.   Female; *age* 55 years; *duration* 1 year; middle finger.

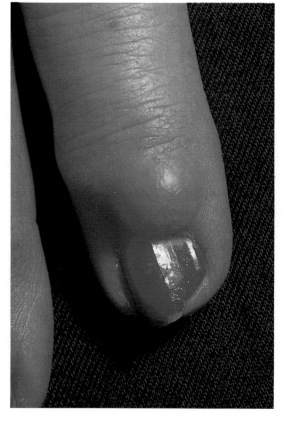

MYXOID DEGENERATION CYST.   Female; *age* 48 years; *duration* 7 months; index finger.

MYXOMA. Female; *age* 53 years; *duration* 9 years; ala nasi; confirmed by biopsy.

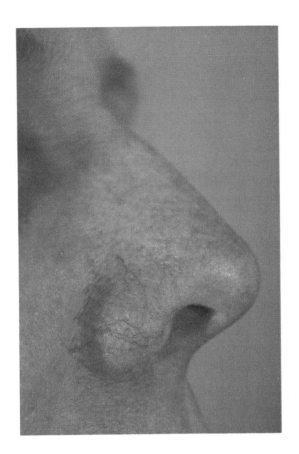

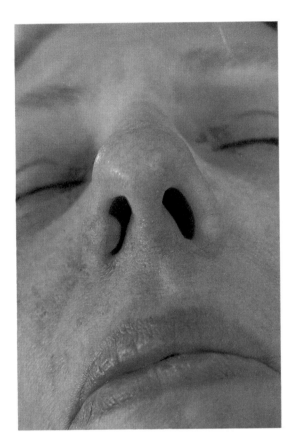

MYXOMA. Female; *age* 53 years; *duration* 9 years; ala nasi; confirmed by biopsy.

MYXOSARCOMA. Female; *age* 49 years; *duration* 15 months; shoulder; confirmed by biopsy. (This tumor metastasized to the axillary lymph nodes.)

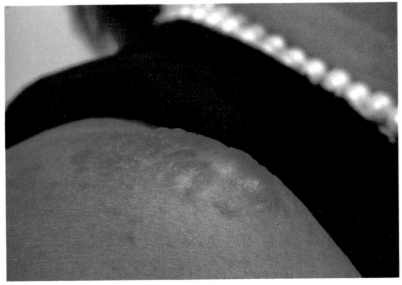

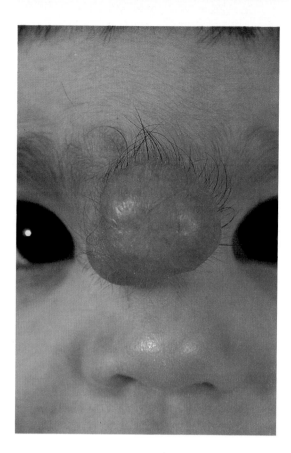

NASAL GLIOMA. Female; *age* 1 year; *duration* since birth; nasal bridge; confirmed by biopsy.

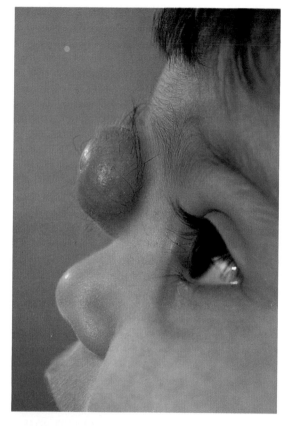

NASAL GLIOMA. Female; *age* 1 year; *duration* since birth; nasal bridge; confirmed by biopsy. (Same patient as in previous photograph.)

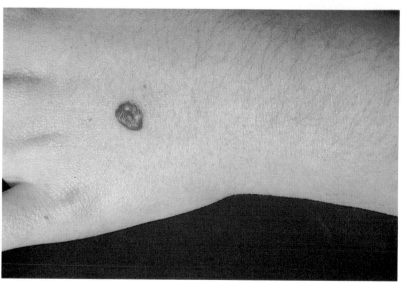

NEVUS, BLUE. Dorsum of hand.

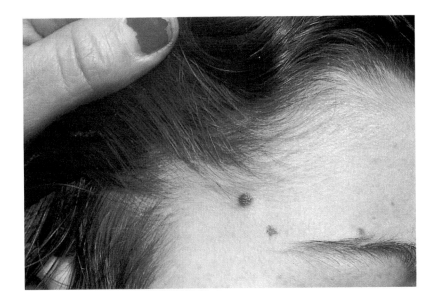

NEVUS, BLUE. Female; *age* 13 years; *duration* since birth; forehead; confirmed by biopsy.

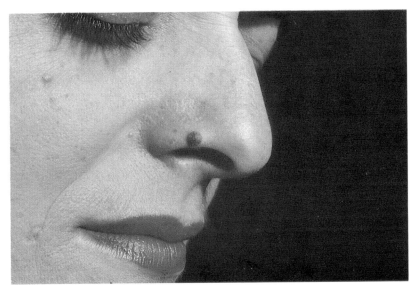

NEVUS, BLUE. Female; *age* unknown; *duration* since birth; nose; confirmed by biopsy.

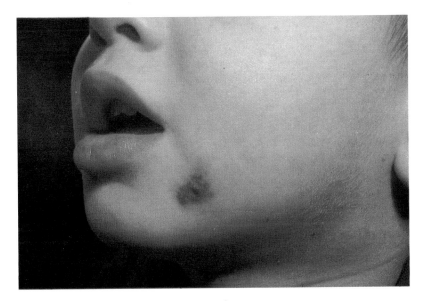

NEVUS, BLUE. Chin.

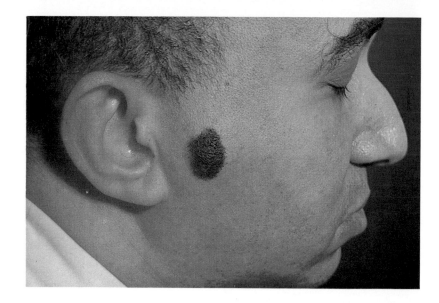

NEVUS, BLUE. Male; *age* 36 years; *duration* since birth; cheek.

NEVUS, BLUE. Female; *age* 49 years; *duration* 15 years; forearm; confirmed by biopsy.

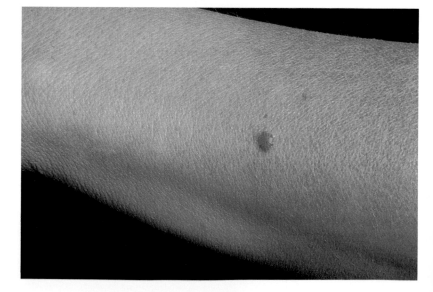

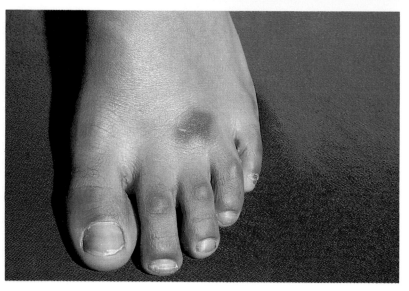

NEVUS, BLUE. Male; *age* 12 years; *duration* 9 years; dorsum of foot.

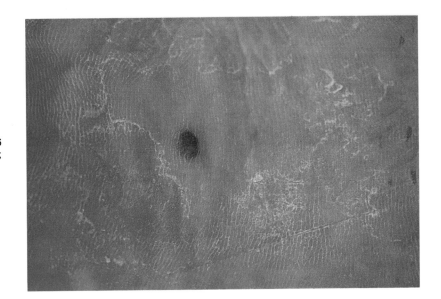

NEVUS, BLUE. Male; *age* 26 years; *duration* since birth; sole.

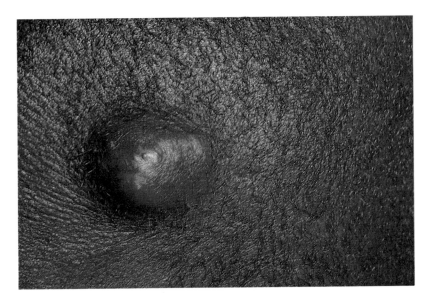

NEURILEMMOMA. Male; *age* 24 years; *duration* 15 years; scalp; confirmed by biopsy.

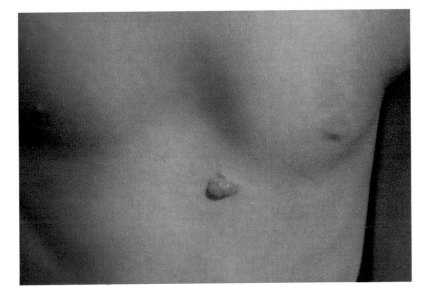

NEUROFIBROMA. Female; *age* 4 years; *duration* since birth; chest; confirmed by biopsy.

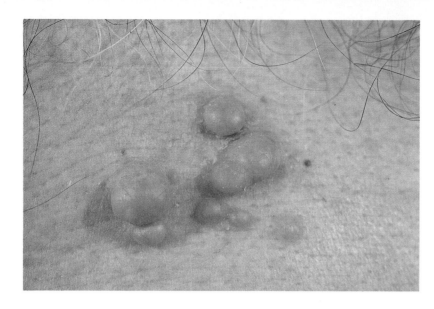

NEUROFIBROMA. Male; *age* 62 years; *duration* 3 years; lower presternal area; confirmed by biopsy.

NEUROFIBROMA. Male; *age* 74 years; upper lip; outer canthus of eye; confirmed by biopsy.

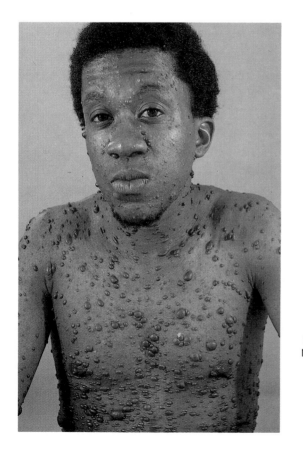

NEUROFIBROMATOSIS. Male; head, neck, trunk, arms.

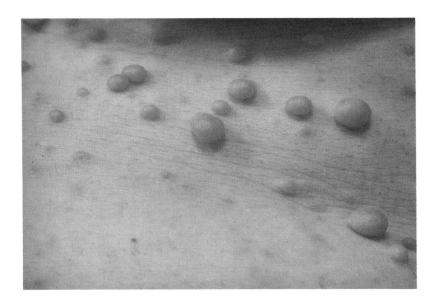

NEUROFIBROMATOSIS. Female; *age* 34 years; trunk.

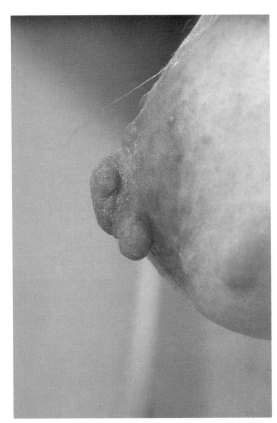

NEUROFIBROMATOSIS. Female; *age* 34 years; breast; confirmed by biopsy.

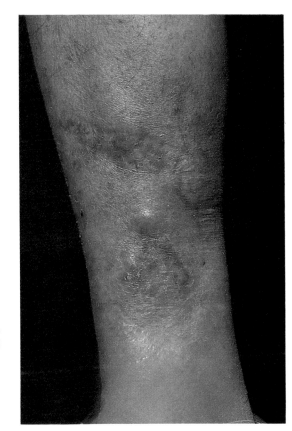

NEUROMA (POSTOPERATIVE). Male; *age* 50 years; leg; confirmed by biopsy.

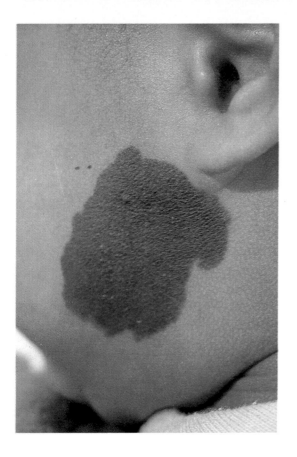

NEVOCYTIC NEVUS (CON-GENITAL). Female; *age* 1 year; *duration* since birth; cheek; confirmed by biopsy.

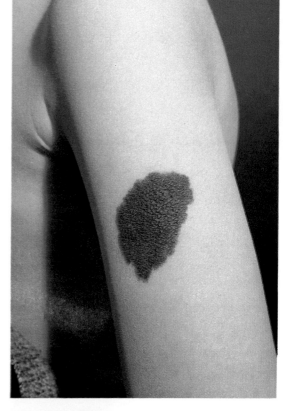

NEVOCYTIC NEVUS (CON-GENITAL). Male; *age* 10 years; *duration* since birth; arm.

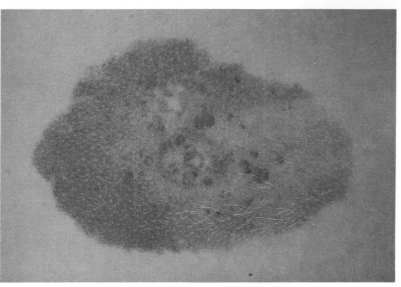

NEVOCYTIC NEVUS (CON-GENITAL). Male; *age* 7 years; *duration* since birth; midback; confirmed by biopsy.

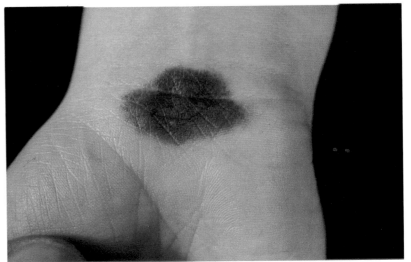

NEVOCYTIC NEVUS (CON-GENITAL). Female; *age* 5 years; *duration* since birth; wrist.

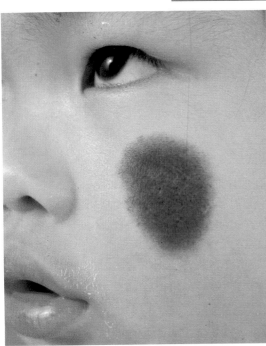

NEVOCYTIC NEVUS (CON-GENITAL). Female; *age* 4 years; *duration* since birth; cheek; confirmed by biopsy.

NEVOCYTIC NEVUS (CON-GENITAL). Male; *age* 6 years; *duration* since birth; chest; confirmed by biopsy.

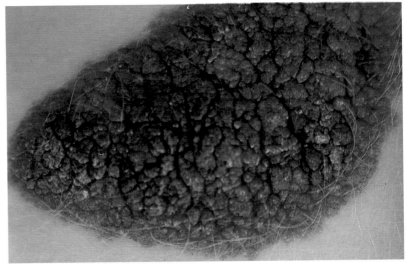

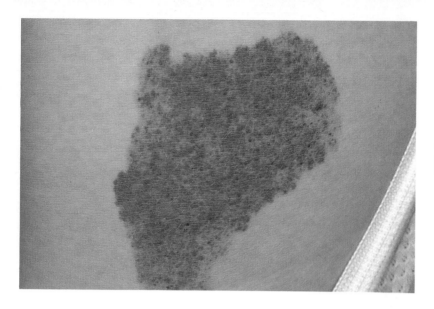

NEVOCYTIC NEVUS (CON-GENITAL). Male; *age* 2 years; hand; confirmed by biopsy.

NEVOCYTIC NEVUS (CON-GENITAL). Female; *age* 9 years; *duration* since birth; lower abdomen; confirmed by biopsy.

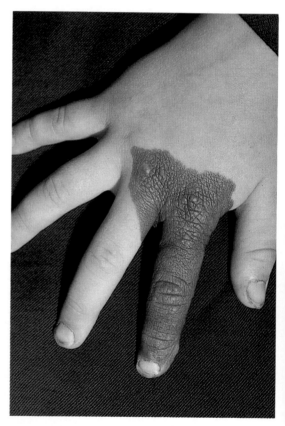

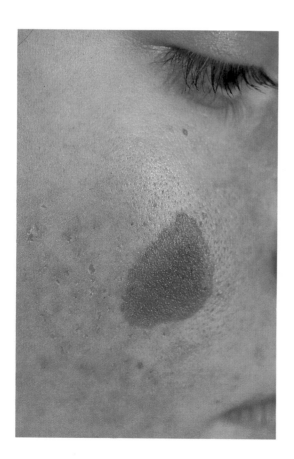

NEVOCYTIC NEVUS (CON-GENITAL). Female; *age* 15 years; *duration* since birth; cheek; confirmed by biopsy.

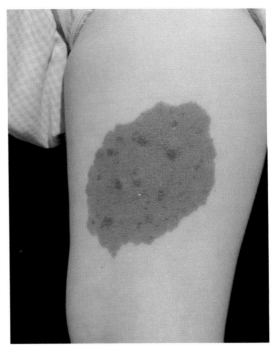

NEVOCYTIC NEVUS (CON-GENITAL). Female; *age* 2 years; *duration* since birth; thigh; confirmed by biopsy.

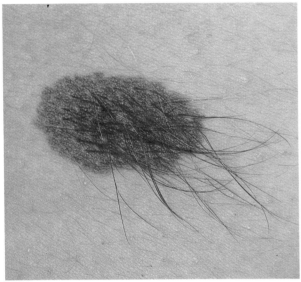

NEVOCYTIC NEVUS (CON-GENITAL). Male; *age* 15 years; back.

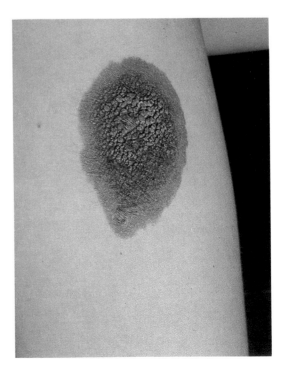

NEVOCYTIC NEVUS (CON-GENITAL). Male; *age* 5 years; *duration* since birth; thigh; confirmed by biopsy.

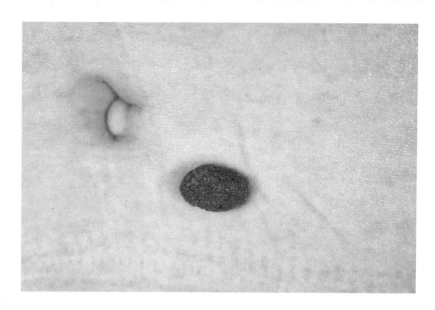

NEVOCYTIC NEVUS (CON-GENITAL). Female; *age* 17 years; *duration* since birth; ab-domen; confirmed by biopsy.

NEVOCYTIC NEVI (CONGEN-ITAL). Female; *age* 17 years; *duration* since birth; lower back; confirmed by biopsy.

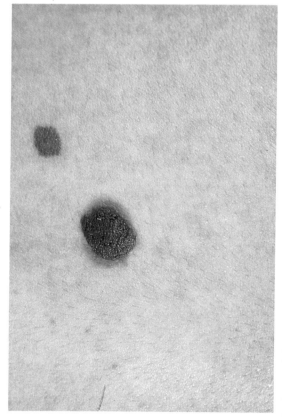

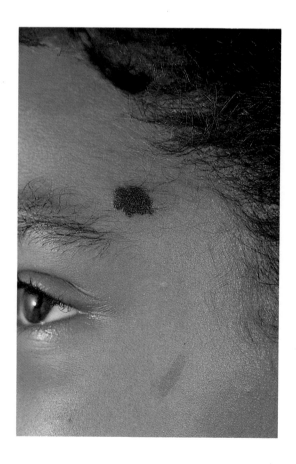

NEVOCYTIC NEVUS (CON-GENITAL). Female; *age* 9 years; *duration* since birth; temple.

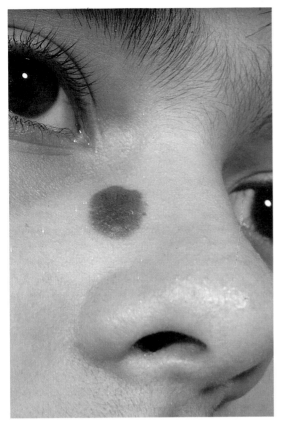

NEVOCYTIC NEVUS (CONGENITAL). Female; *age* 6 years; *duration* since birth; nose; confirmed by biopsy.

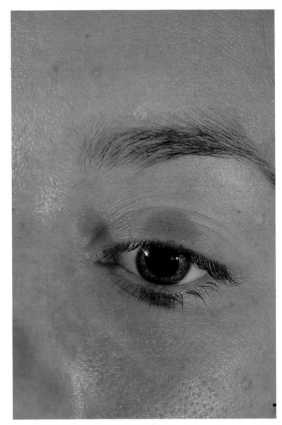

NEVOCYTIC NEVUS (DIVIDED). Female; *age* 18 years; *duration* since birth; eyelids.

NEVOCYTIC NEVUS (CONGENITAL). Female; *age* 24 years; *duration* since birth; leg; confirmed by biopsy.

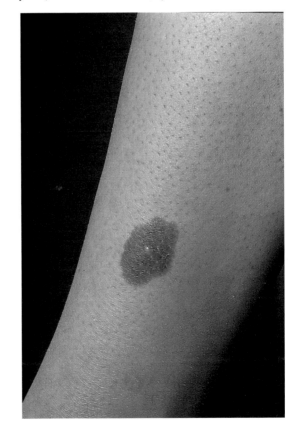

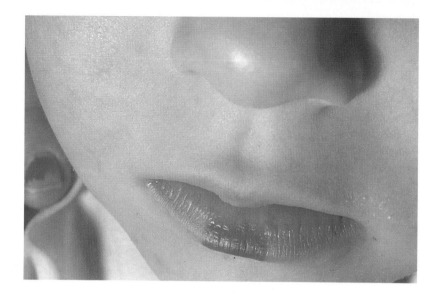

NEVOCYTIC NEVUS (CON-GENITAL). Female; *age* 5 years; *duration* since birth; lower lip.

NEVOCYTIC NEVUS. Female; *age* 16 years; *duration* 11 years; breast.

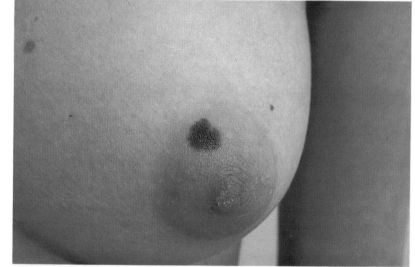

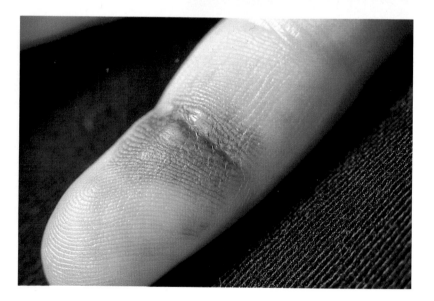

NEVOCYTIC NEVUS (CON-GENITAL). Female; *age* 8 years; *duration* since birth; finger; confirmed by biopsy.

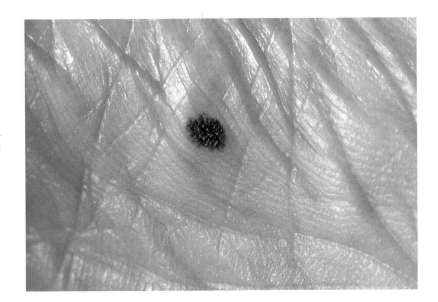

NEVOCYTIC NEVUS. Female; *age* 31 years; sole; confirmed by biopsy.

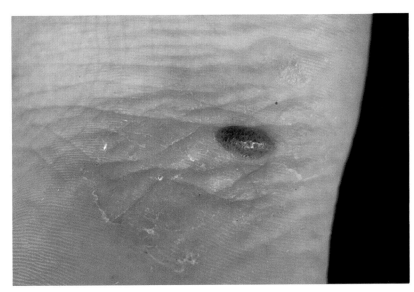

NEVOCYTIC NEVUS (CONGENITAL). Male; *age* 13 years; *duration* since birth; sole; confirmed by biopsy.

NEVOCYTIC NEVUS (CONGENITAL). Female; *age* 29 years; *duration* since birth; breast; confirmed by biopsy.

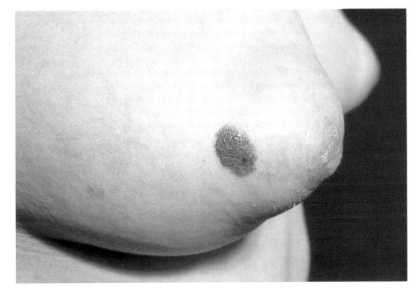

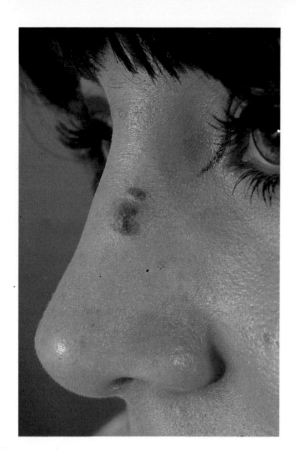

NEVUS-CELL NEVUS. Female; *age* 20 years; *duration* since birth; nose; confirmed by biopsy.

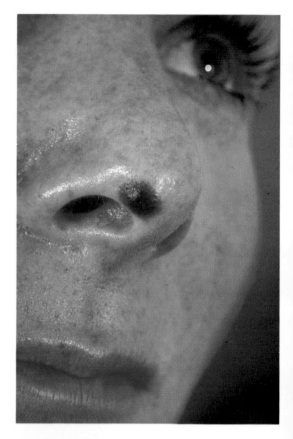

NEVOCYTIC NEVUS. Female; *age* 25 years; *duration* 3 years; nose.

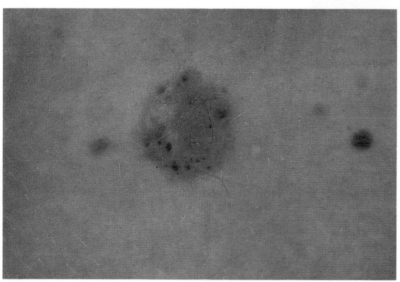

NEVOCYTIC NEVUS. Male; *age* 16 years; *duration* 7 years; back; confirmed by biopsy.

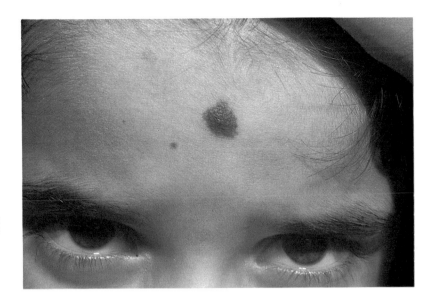

NEVOCYTIC NEVUS. Male; *age* 7 years; *duration* since birth; forehead.

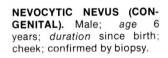

NEVOCYTIC NEVUS (CON-GENITAL). Male; *age* 6 years; *duration* since birth; cheek; confirmed by biopsy.

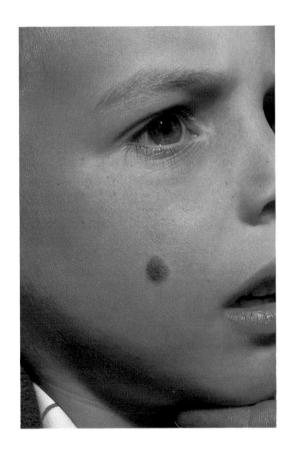

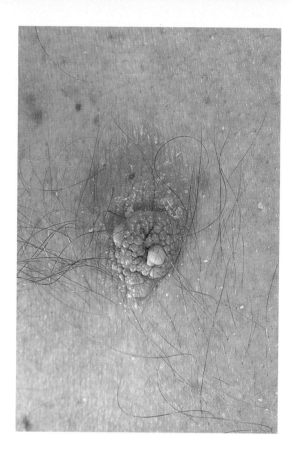

NEVOCYTIC NEVUS (CON-GENITAL). Male; *age* 35 years; *duration* since birth; back; confirmed by biopsy.

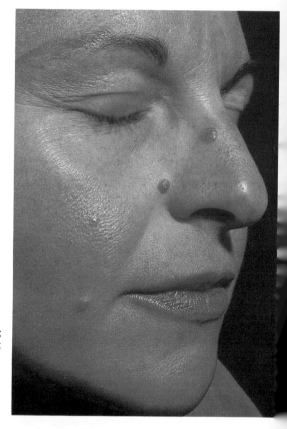

NEVOCYTIC NEVI. Female; *age* 40 years; *duration* 5 years; face.

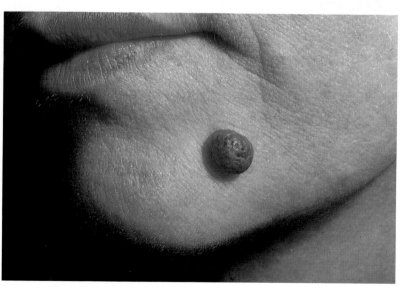

NEVOCYTIC NEVUS. Female; *age* 38 years; *duration* since birth; chin; confirmed by biopsy.

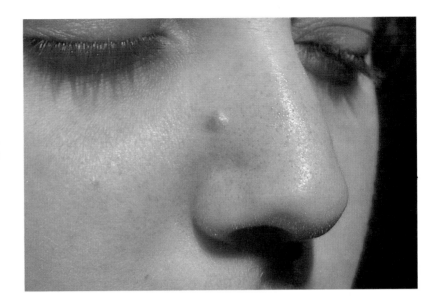

NEVOCYTIC NEVUS. Female; *age* 24 years; *duration* 4 years; nose.

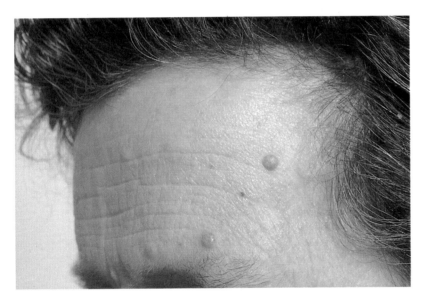

NEVOCYTIC NEVI. Female; *age* 57 years; forehead; confirmed by biopsy.

NEVOCYTIC NEVUS. Female; *age* 36 years; *duration* since birth; cheek; confirmed by biopsy.

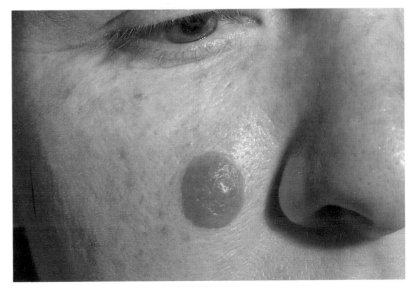

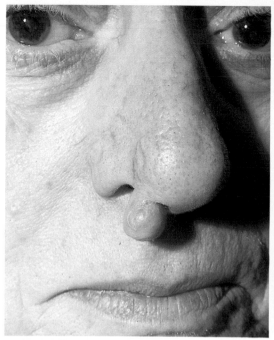

NEVOCYTIC NEVUS. Male; *age* 74 years; *duration* 9 years; nose; confirmed by biopsy.

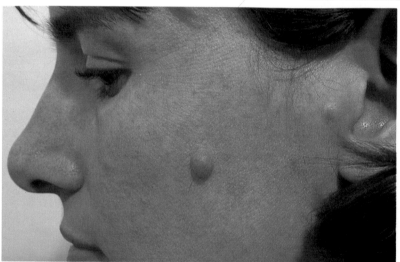

NEVOCYTIC NEVUS. Female; *age* 29 years; *duration* 12 years; cheek; confirmed by biopsy.

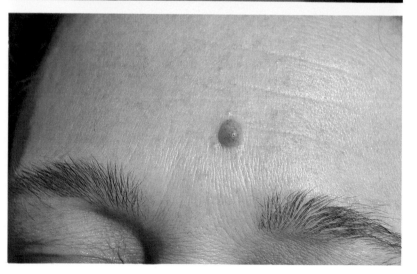

NEVOCYTIC NEVUS. Female; *age* 53 years; *duration* since birth; forehead; confirmed by biopsy.

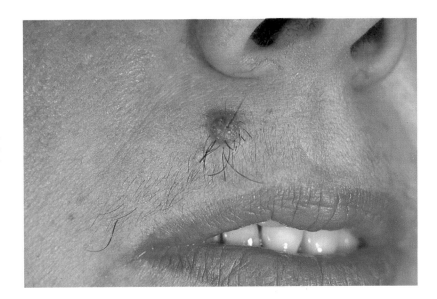

NEVOCYTIC NEVUS. Female; *age* 39 years; *duration* since birth; upper lip; confirmed by biopsy.

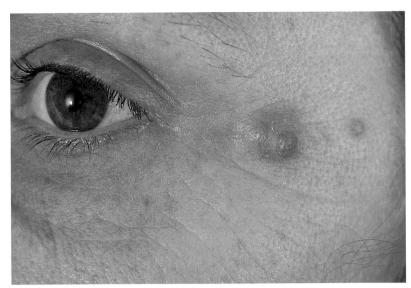

NEVOCYTIC NEVUS (WITH UNDERLYING CYST). Female; temple.

NEVOCYTIC NEVUS. Male; *age* 15 years; *duration* 14 years; cheek.

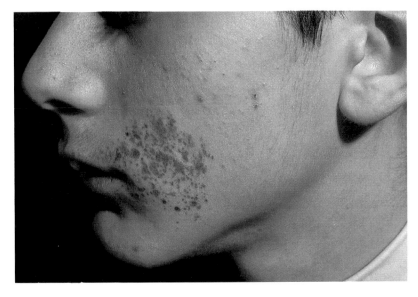

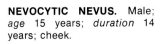

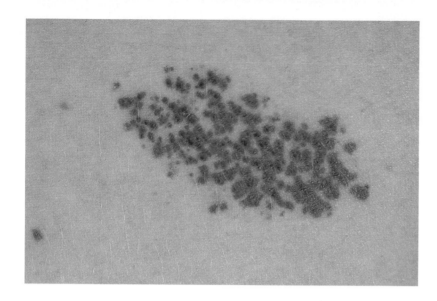

NEVOCYTIC NEVUS. Male; *age* 15 years; *duration* since birth; back; confirmed by biopsy.

NEVOCYTIC NEVUS. Female; *age* 9 years; *duration* since birth; cheek.

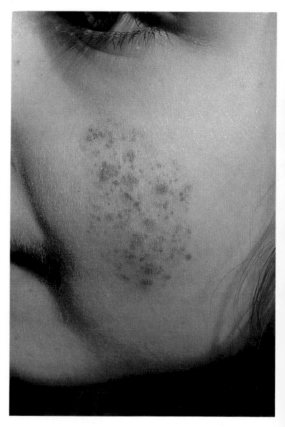

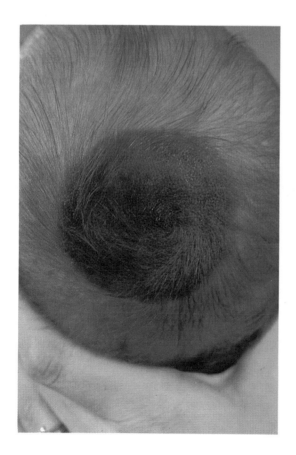

NEVOCYTIC NEVUS (CONGENITAL). Male; *age* 7 weeks; *duration* since birth; scalp.

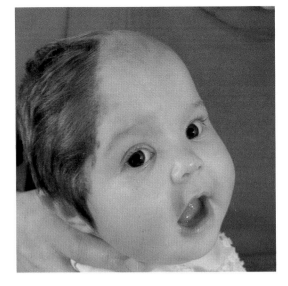

NEVOCYTIC NEVUS (CON-GENITAL). Female; *age* 14 weeks; *duration* since birth; scalp; confirmed by biopsy.

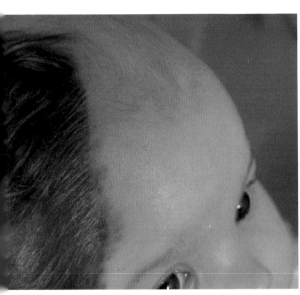

NEVOCYTIC NEVUS (CON-GENITAL). Female; *age* 14 weeks; *duration* since birth; scalp; confirmed by biopsy. (Same patient as in previous photograph.)

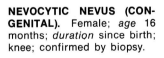

NEVOCYTIC NEVUS (CON-GENITAL). Female; *age* 16 months; *duration* since birth; knee; confirmed by biopsy.

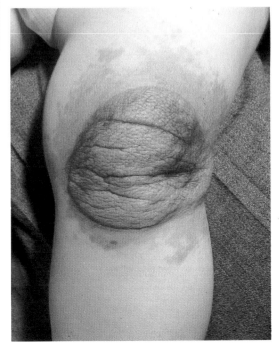

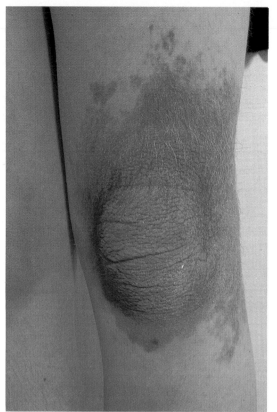

NEVOCYTIC NEVUS (CONGENITAL). Female; *age* 7 years; *duration* since birth; knee; confirmed by biopsy. (Same patient as in previous photograph.)

NEVOCYTIC NEVUS (CONGENITAL). Female; *age* 8 years; *duration* since birth; knee; confirmed by biopsy. (Same patient as in previous photograph.)

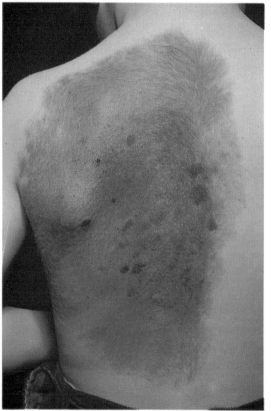

NEVOCYTIC NEVUS (CONGENITAL). Male; *age* 5 years; *duration* since birth; back.

NEVOCYTIC NEVUS (CON-GENITAL). Female; *age* 1 month; *duration* since birth; thigh.

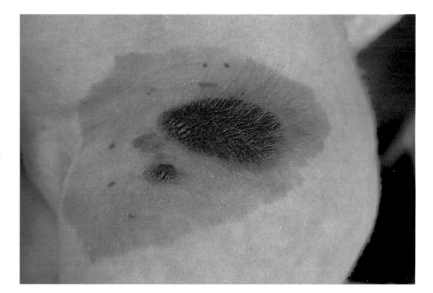

NEVOCYTIC NEVUS (CON-GENITAL). Male; *duration* since birth; leg; confirmed by biopsy.

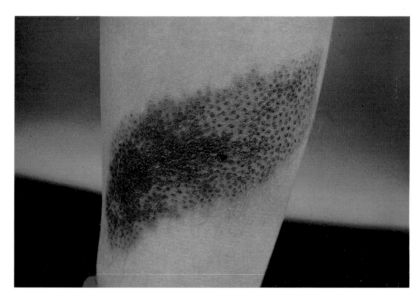

NEVOCYTIC NEVUS (CON-GENITAL). Male; *age* 3 years; *duration* since birth; back.

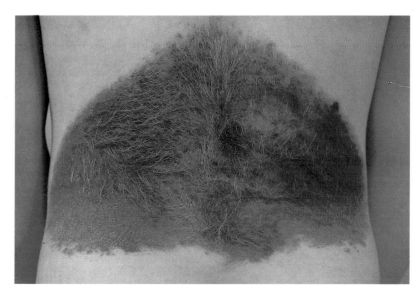

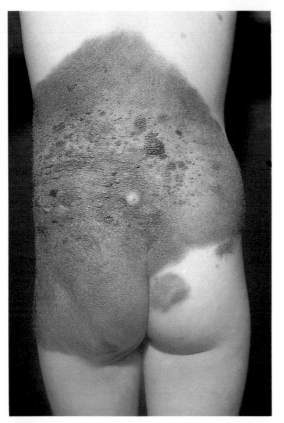

NEVOCYTIC NEVUS (CONGENITAL). Buttocks and back.

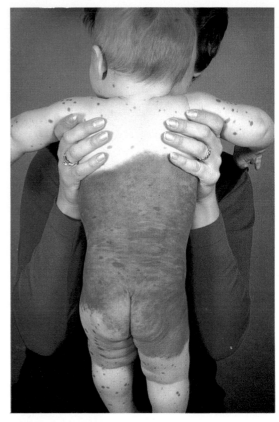

NEVOCYTIC NEVUS (CONGENITAL). Male; infant; trunk and extremities.

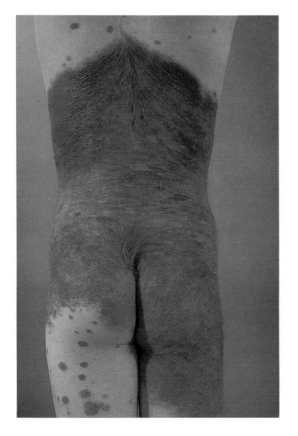

NEVOCYTIC NEVUS (CONGENITAL). Male; *age* 5 years; *duration* since birth; trunk and thighs. (Same patient as in previous photograph.)

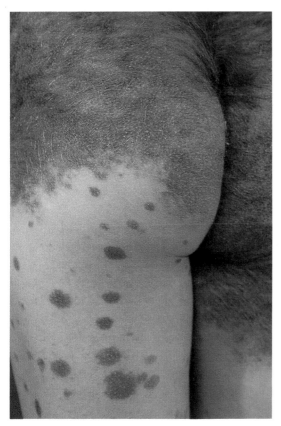

NEVOCYTIC NEVUS (CONGENITAL). Male; *age* 5 years; *duration* since birth; buttocks and thighs. (Same patient as in previous photograph.)

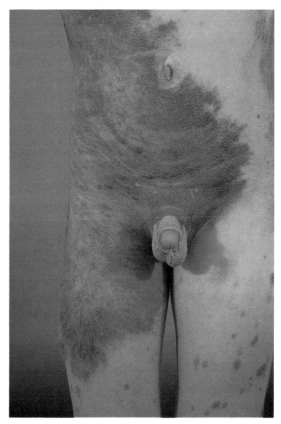

NEVOCYTIC NEVUS (CONGENITAL). Male; *age* 5 years; *duration* since birth; trunk and thighs. (Same patient as in previous photograph.)

NEVOCYTIC NEVUS (CONGENITAL). Male; *age* 3 months; *duration* since birth; face.

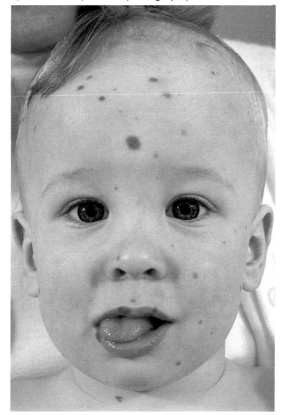

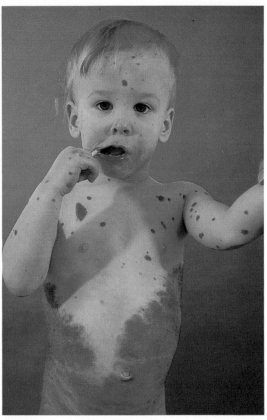

NEVOCYTIC NEVUS (CONGENITAL). Male; *age* 12 months; *duration* since birth; face, trunk and upper extremities. (Same patient as in previous photograph.)

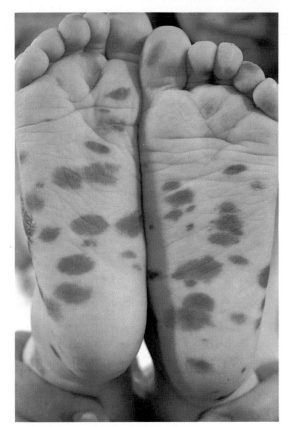

NEVOCYTIC NEVUS (CONGENITAL). Male; *age* 3 months; *duration* since birth; soles. (Same patient as in previous photograph.)

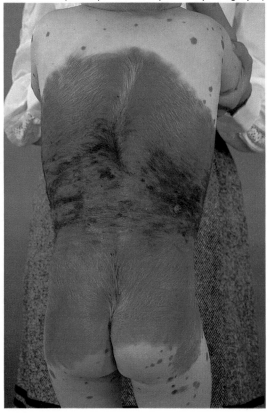

NEVOCYTIC NEVUS (CONGENITAL). Male; *age* 6 months; *duration* since birth; trunk; confirmed by biopsy. (Same patient as in previous photograph.)

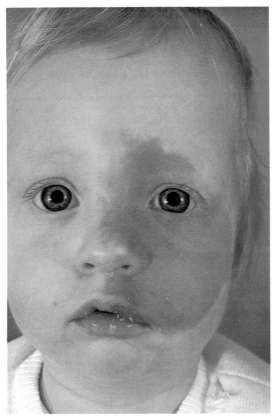

NEVUS FLAMMEUS. Female; *age* 1 year; *duration* since birth; face.

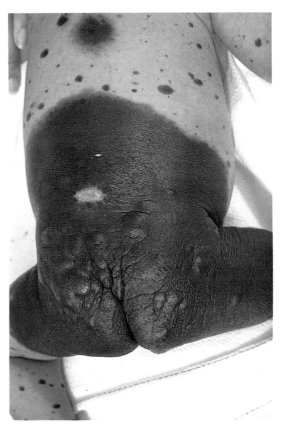

NEVOCYTIC NEVUS (CONGENITAL). Male; trunk, buttocks and thighs.

NEVUS FLAMMEUS. Male; *duration* since birth; face.

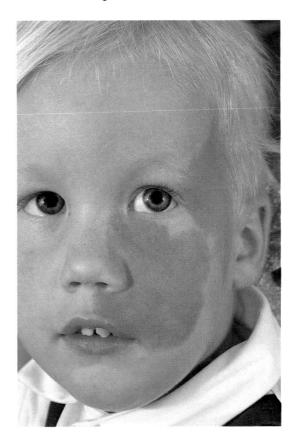

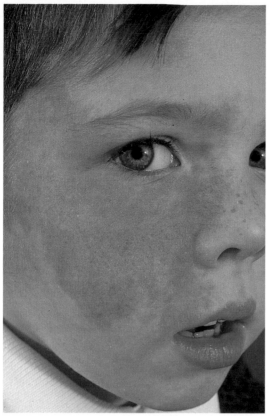

NEVUS FLAMMEUS. Male; *age* 1 year; *duration* since birth; cheek; forehead, temple and upper lip.

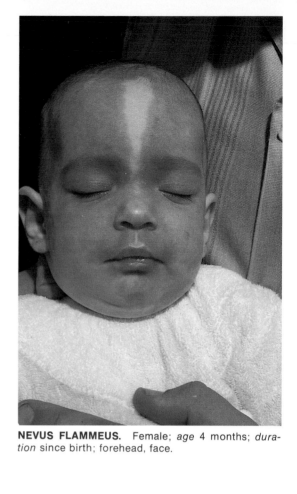

NEVUS FLAMMEUS. Female; *age* 4 months; *duration* since birth; forehead, face.

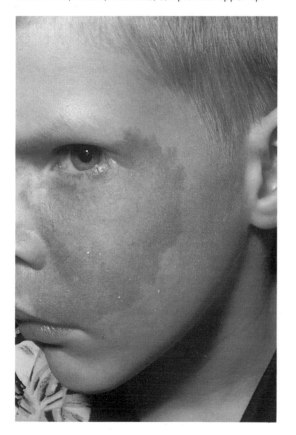

NEVUS FLAMMEUS. Male; *age* 14 years; *duration* since birth; face.

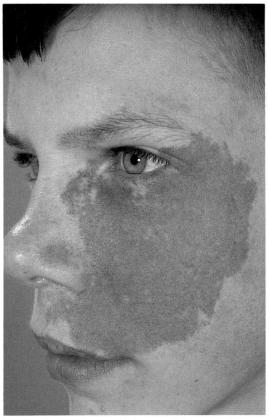

NEVUS FLAMMEUS. Male; *age* 14 years; *duration* since birth; cheek, upper lip, nose, eyelids. (Same patient as in previous photograph.)

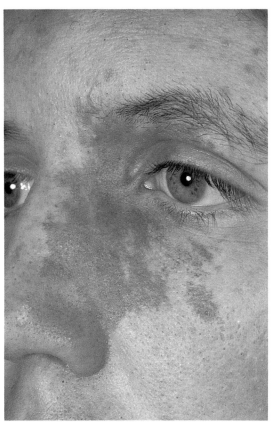

NEVUS FLAMMEUS. Male; *age* 17 years; *duration* since birth; eyelids, nose and paranasal area.

NEVUS FLAMMEUS (STURGE-WEBER). Male; *duration* since birth; forehead and temple.

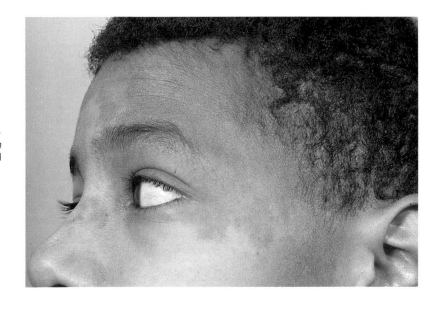

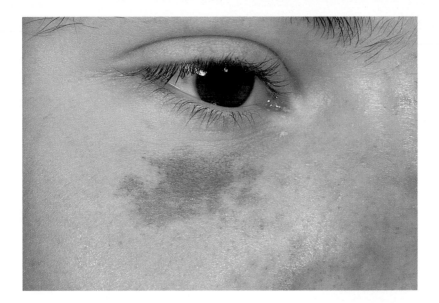

NEVUS FLAMMEUS. Male; *age* 15 years; *duration* since birth; lower eyelid and cheek.

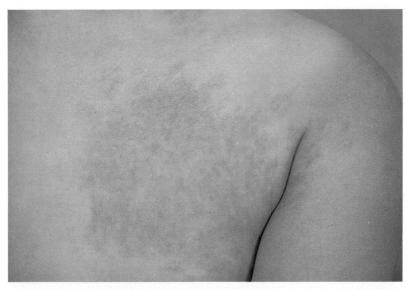

NEVUS FLAMMEUS. Female; *age* 3 years; *duration* since birth; chest.

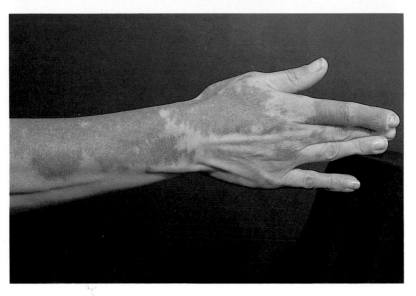

NEVUS FLAMMEUS. Female; *age* 39 years; forearm and hand.

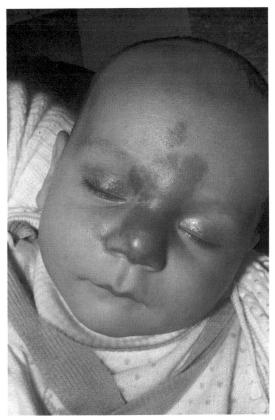

NAVUS FLAMMEUS. Male; *age* 3 months; *duration* since birth; forehead, eyelid, nose; confirmed by biopsy.

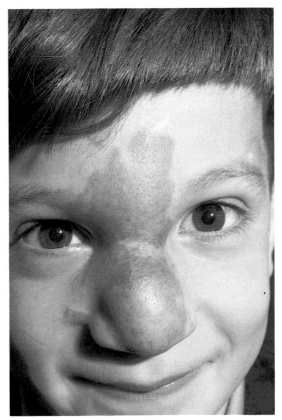

NEVUS FLAMMEUS. Male; *age* 7 years; *duration* since birth; forehead, nose. (Same patient as in previous photograph.)

NEVUS FLAMMEUS (HYPERTROPHIC). Male; *age* 65 years; *duration* since birth; nose, upper eyelid.

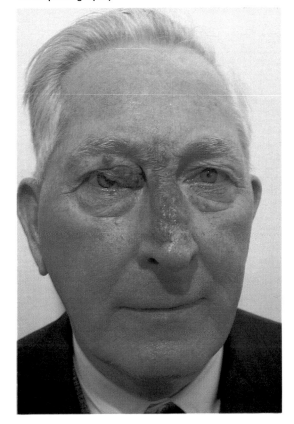

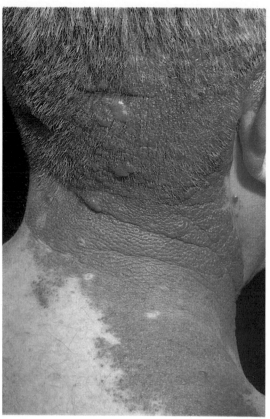

NEVUS FLAMMEUS (HYPERTROPHIC). Male; *age* 28 years; *duration* since birth; head and neck; confirmed by biopsy.

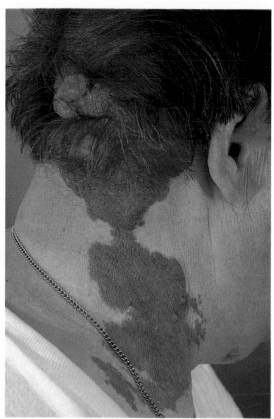

NEVUS FLAMMEUS (HYPERTROPHIC). Female; *age* 51 years; *duration* since birth; occipital and cervical areas; confirmed by biopsy.

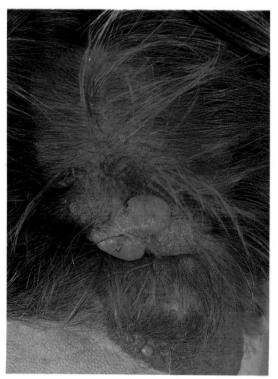

NEVUS FLAMMEUS (HYPERTROPHIC). Female; *age* 51 years; *duration* since birth; occipital and cervical areas; confirmed by biopsy. (Same patient as in previous photograph.)

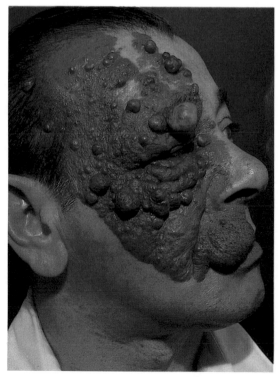

NEVUS FLAMMEUS (HYPERTROPHIC). Male; *age* 50 years; *duration* since birth; scalp, forehead and face.

NEVUS SEBACEUS. Female; *age* 4 years; *duration* since birth; scalp; confirmed by biopsy.

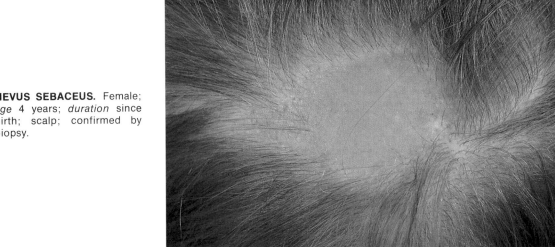

NEVUS SEBACEUS. Male; *age* 2 years; *duration* since birth; scalp.

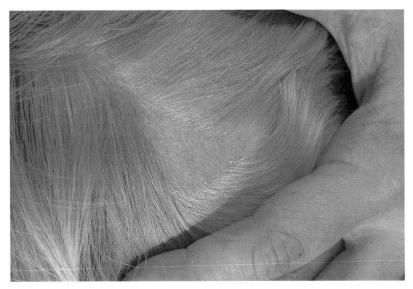

NEVUS SEBACEUS. Male; *age* 10 months; *duration* since birth; forehead.

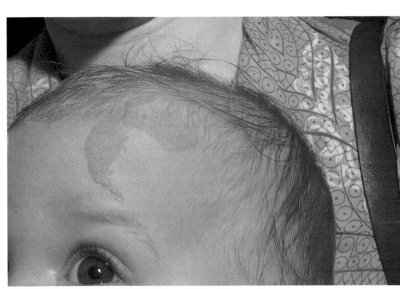

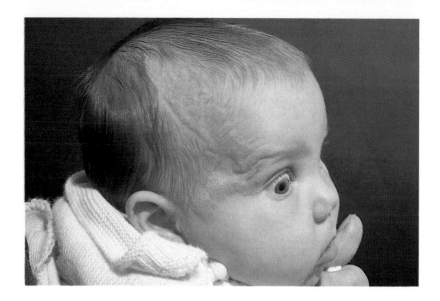

NEVUS SEBACEUS. Female; *age* 5 months; *duration* since birth; scalp and temple; confirmed by biopsy.

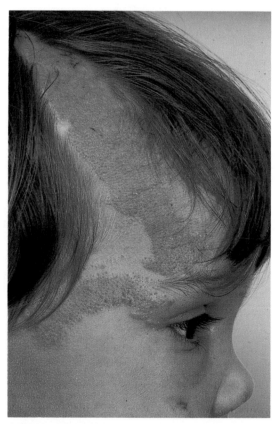

NEVUS SEBACEUS. Female; *age* 2 years; *duration* since birth; scalp and temple; confirmed by biopsy. (Same patient as in previous photograph.)

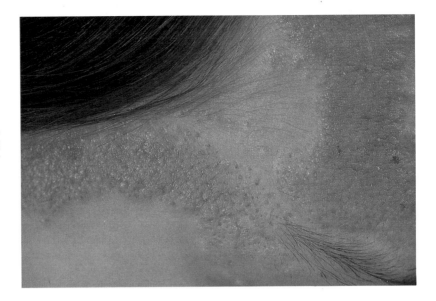

NEVUS SEBACEUS. Female; *duration* since birth; forehead and temple; confirmed by biopsy.

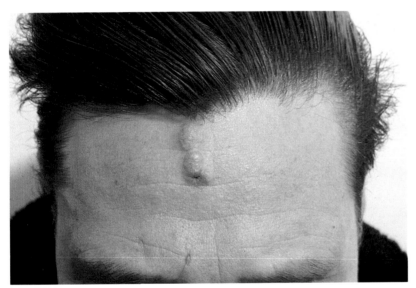

NEVUS SEBACEUS. Male; *age* 43 years; forehead; confirmed by biopsy.

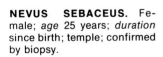

NEVUS SEBACEUS. Female; *age* 25 years; *duration* since birth; temple; confirmed by biopsy.

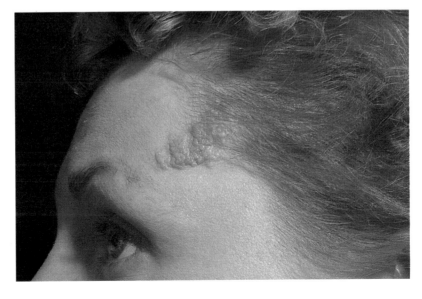

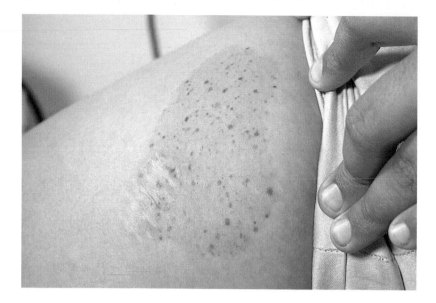

NEVUS SPILUS. Male; *age* 15 years; *duration* since birth; thigh; confirmed by biopsy.

NEVUS SPILUS. Female; cheek.

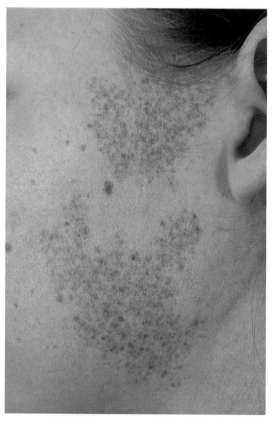

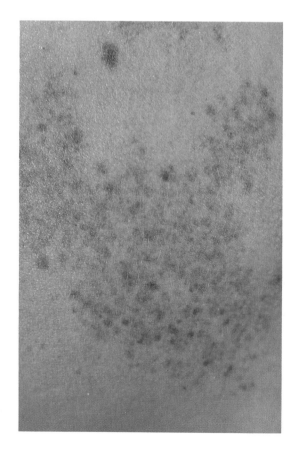

NEVUS SPILUS. Female; cheek. (Same patient as in previous photograph.)

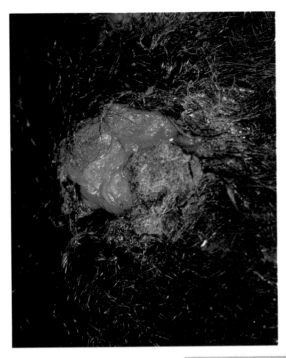

**NEVUS SYRINGOCYSTA-
DENOMATOSUS PAPILLI-
FERUS (WERTHER).** Male;
age teens; scalp; confirmed by
biopsy.

NEVUS UNIUS LATERIS. Female; *age* 5 years; neck.

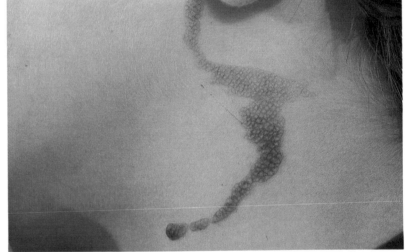

NEVUS UNIUS LATERIS.
Male; *age* 8 years; *duration*
since birth; abdomen; confirmed by biopsy.

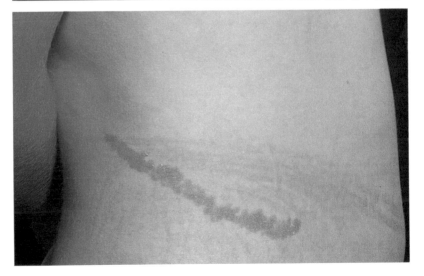

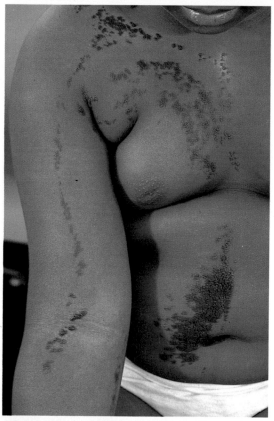

NEVUS UNIUS LATERIS. Female; *age* 8 years; trunk and upper extremity.

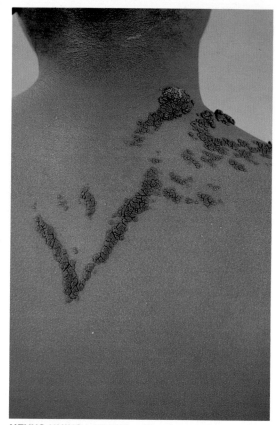

NEVUS UNIUS LATERIS. Female; *age* 8 years; back. (Same patient as in previous photograph.)

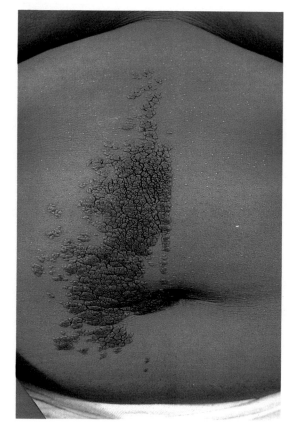

NEVUS UNIUS LATERIS. Female; *age* 8 years; abdomen.

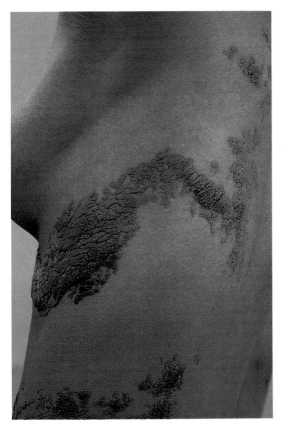

NEVUS UNIUS LATERIS. Female; trunk.

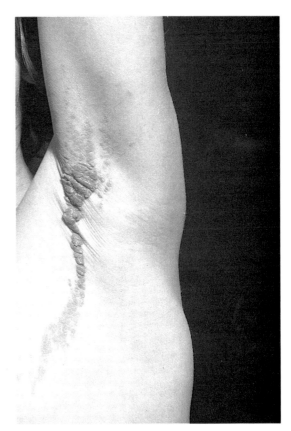

NEVUS UNIUS LATERIS. Female; *age* 6 years; *duration* over 5 years; axilla and chest; confirmed by biopsy.

NEVUS UNIUS LATERIS. Female; face.

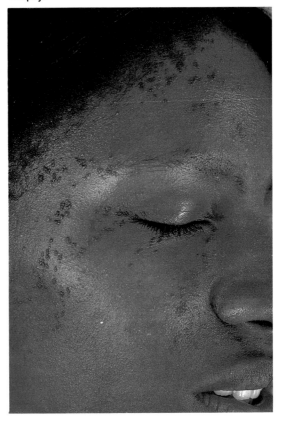

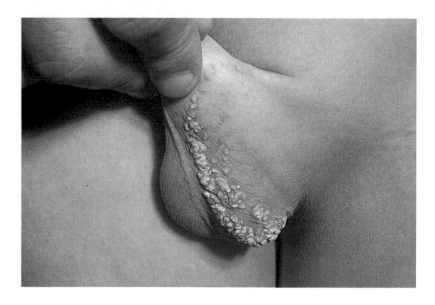

NEVUS UNIUS LATERIS.
Male; *age* 9 years; *duration* 5 years; scrotum; confirmed by biopsy.

NEVUS UNIUS LATERIS.
Male; *age* 16 years; *duration* 7 years; hand and forearm.

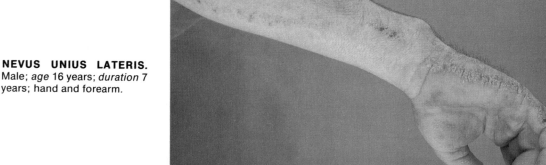

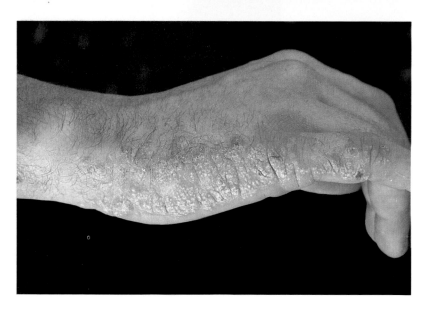

NEVUS UNIUS LATERIS.
Male; *age* 16 years; *duration* 7 years; hand. (Same patient as in previous photograph.)

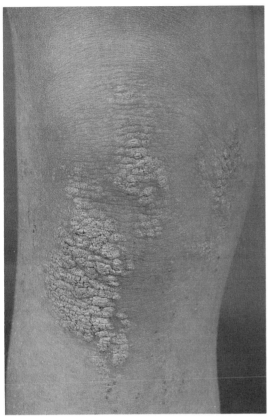

NEVUS UNIUS LATERIS. Female; *age* 4 years; *duration* since birth; knee.

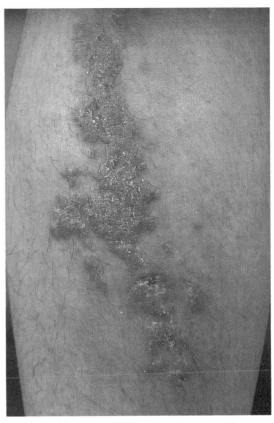

NEVUS UNIUS LATERIS. Female; *age* 13 years; *duration* 4 years; leg; confirmed by biopsy.

NEVUS UNIUS LATERIS. Male; *age* 25 years; abdomen.

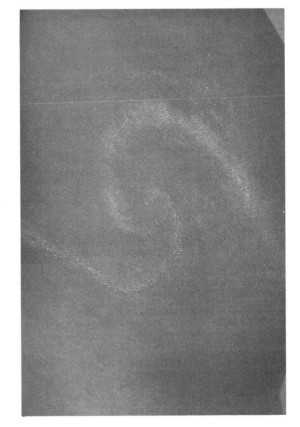

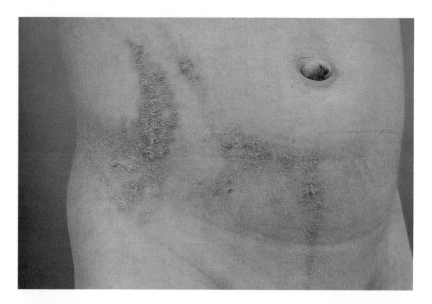

NEVUS UNIUS LATERIS. Female; *age* 4 years; *duration* since birth; abdomen.

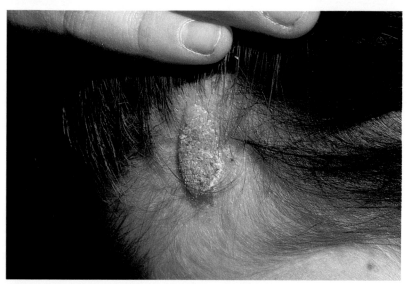

NEVUS VERRUCOSUS. Female; *age* 10 years; *duration* since birth; scalp; confirmed by biopsy.

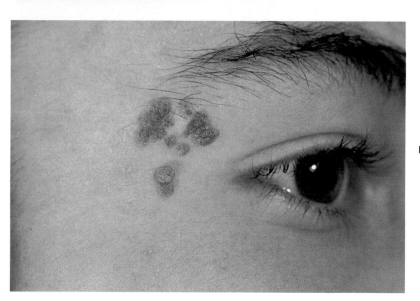

NEVUS VERRUCOSUS. Temple

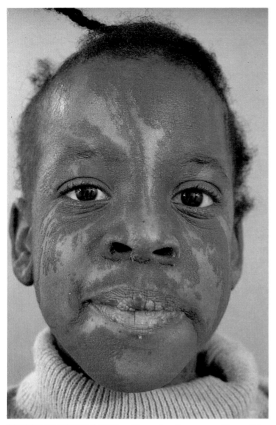

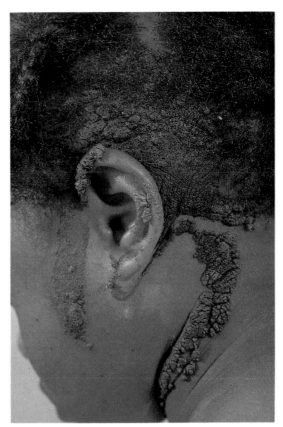

NEVUS VERRUCOSUS. Female; face; confirmed by biopsy.

NEVUS VERRUCOSUS. Female; face, neck, ear and scalp; confirmed by biopsy.

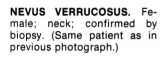

NEVUS VERRUCOSUS. Female; neck; confirmed by biopsy. (Same patient as in previous photograph.)

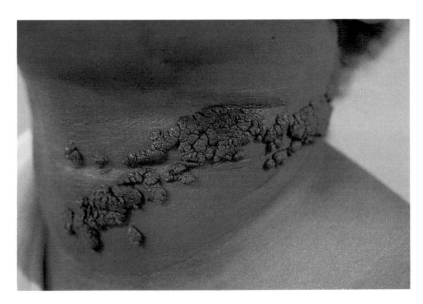

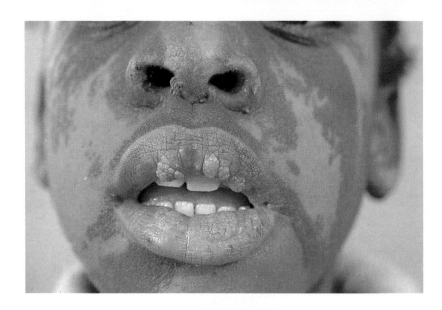

NEVUS VERRUCOSUS. Female; face; confirmed by biopsy. (Same patient as in previous photograph.)

NODULUS CUTANEUS. Male; *age* 45 years; *duration* 5 years; leg; confirmed by biopsy.

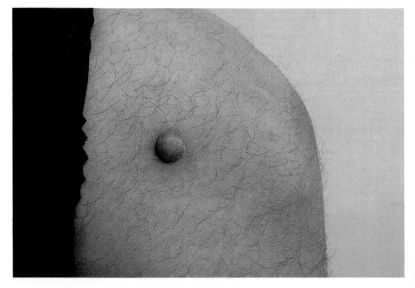

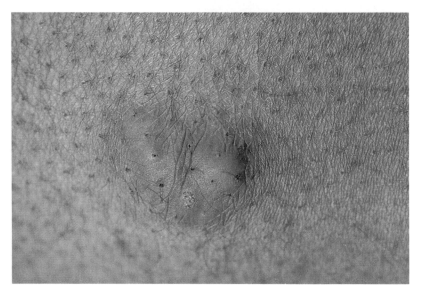

NODULUS CUTANEUS. Female; *age* 20 years; thigh.

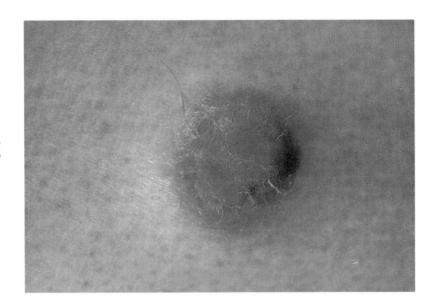

NODULUS CUTANEUS. Female; *age* 41 years; *duration* 5 years; leg.

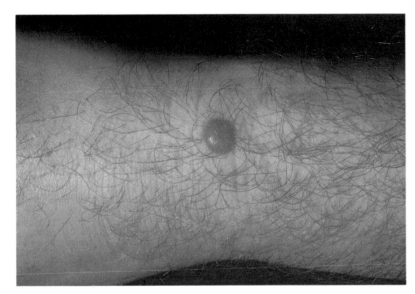

NODULUS CUTANEUS. Male; *age* 49 years; *duration* 3 years; wrist; confirmed by biopsy.

NODULUS CUTANEUS. Female; *age* 31 years; *duration* 3 years; back; confirmed by biopsy.

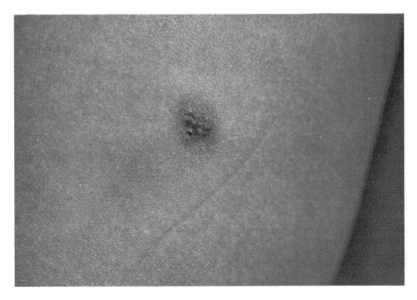

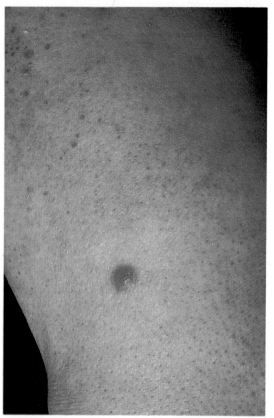

NODULUS CUTANEUS. Male; *age* 68 years; *duration* 2 years; leg; confirmed by biopsy.

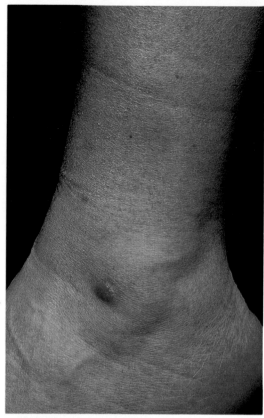

NODULUS CUTANEUS. Male; *age* 45 years; *duration* 10 years; ankle; confirmed by biopsy.

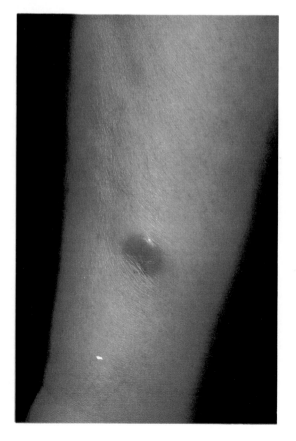

NODULUS CUTANEUS. Female; *age* 70 years; *duration* 35 years; leg; confirmed by biopsy.

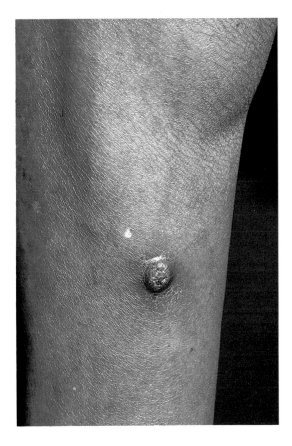

NODULUS CUTANEUS.
Male; *age* 46 years; *duration* 12 years; leg; confirmed by biopsy.

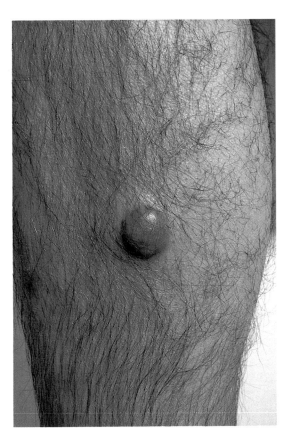

NODULUS CUTANEUS.
Male; *age* 27 years; *duration* 17 years; leg; confirmed by biopsy.

NODULUS CUTANEUS.
Male; *age* 65 years; *duration* 25 years; arm; confirmed by biopsy.

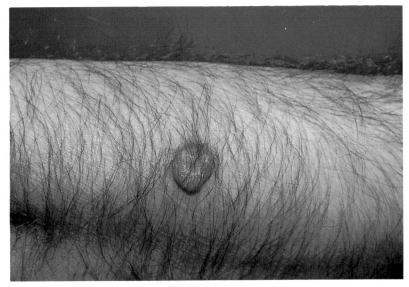

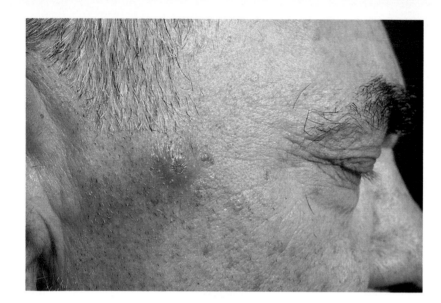

ONCOCYTOMA. Male; *age* 71 years; *duration* 4 years; temple; confirmed by biopsy.

ORAL FLORID PAPILLOMA-TOSIS. Male; *age* 63 years; *duration* 13 months; lower lip; confirmed by biopsy.

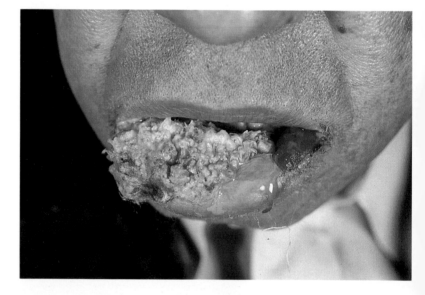

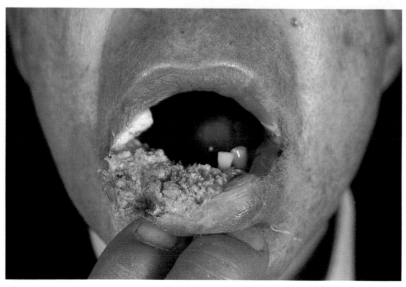

ORAL FLORID PAPILLOMA-TOSIS. Male; *age* 63 years; *duration* 13 months; lower lip; confirmed by biopsy. (Same patient as in previous photograph.)

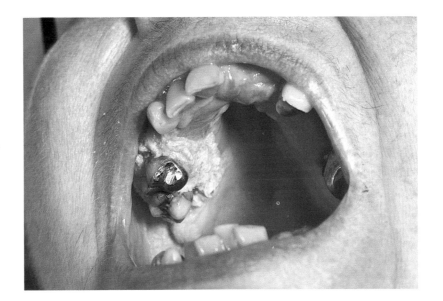

ORAL FLORID PAPILLOMA-TOSIS. Female; gingiva.

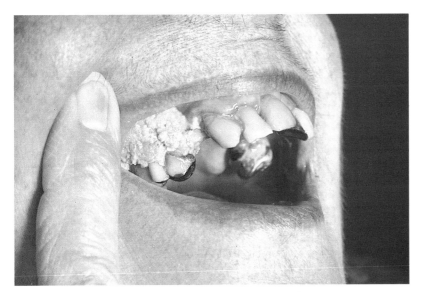

ORAL FLORID PAPILLOMA-TOSIS. Female; gingiva. (Same patient as in previous photograph.)

OSTEOMA (SUBUNGUAL). Male; *age* 56 years; *duration* 12 years; finger.

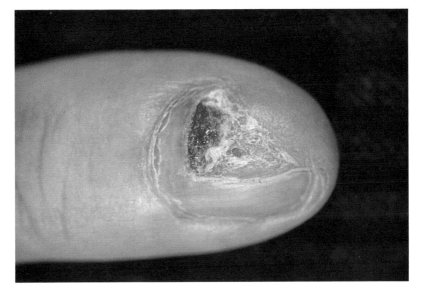

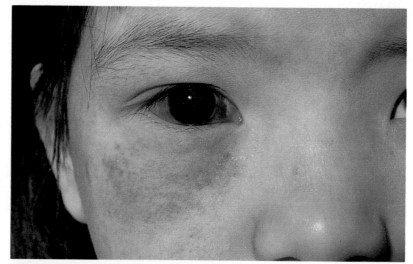

OTA'S NEVUS. Male; *age* 6 years; *duration* since birth; eyelid and sclera.

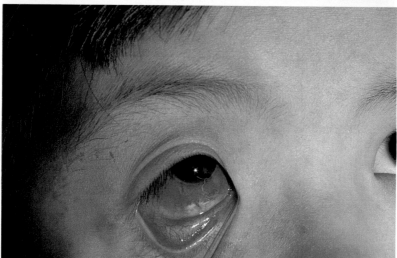

OTA'S NEVUS. Male; *age* 6 years; *duration* since birth. (Same patient as in previous photograph.)

OTA'S NEVUS. Female; *age* 33 years; *duration* since birth; cheek.

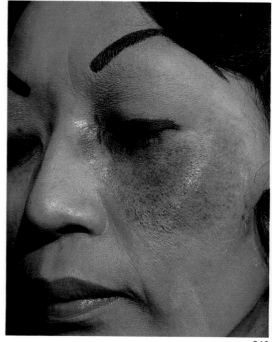

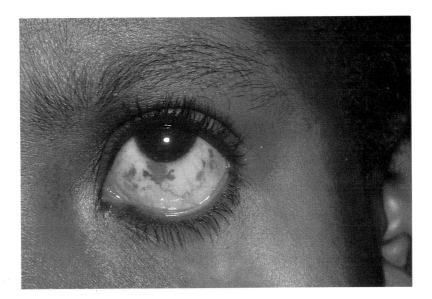

OTA'S NEVUS. Female; *age* 7 years; *duration* since birth; sclera; confirmed by biopsy.

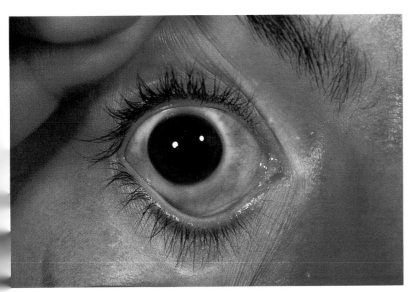

OTA'S NEVUS. Male; *age* 16 years; *duration* since birth; sclera.

PAGET'S DISEASE OF BREAST. Female; breast.

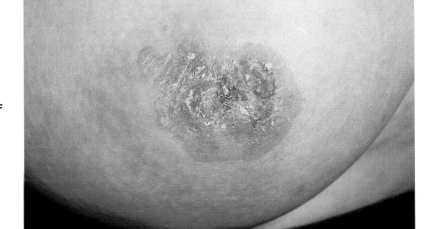

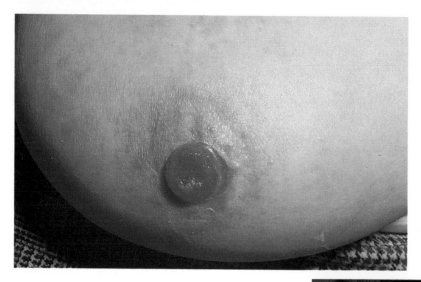

PAGET'S DISEASE OF BREAST. Female; *age* 66 years; *duration* 5 months; nipple.

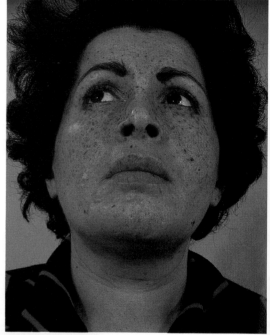

PEUTZ - JEGHERS SYN-DROME. Female; *age* 41 years; *duration* since birth; face and lips.

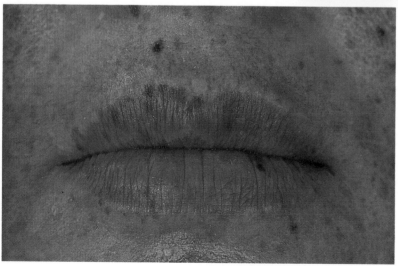

PEUTZ - JEGHERS SYN-DROME. Female; *age* 41 years; *duration* since birth; face and lips. (Same patient as in previous photograph.)

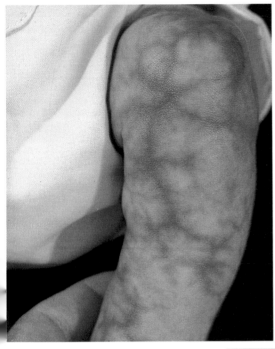

PHLEBECTASIA. Male; *infant*; lower extremity.

PHLEBECTASIA. Female; *age* 69 years; *duration* 49 years; finger; confirmed by biopsy.

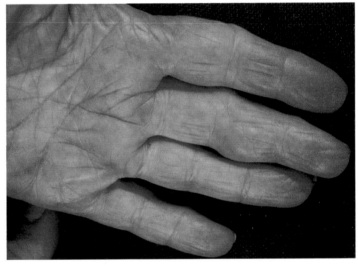

PILOMATRICOMA. Female; *age* 10 years; *duration* 5 months; arm; confirmed by biopsy.

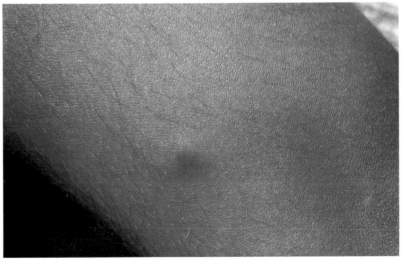

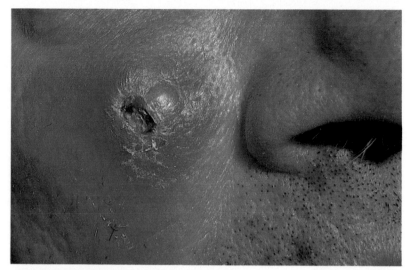

PILOMATRICOMA. Male; *age* 69 years; *duration* 3 months; cheek; confirmed by biopsy.

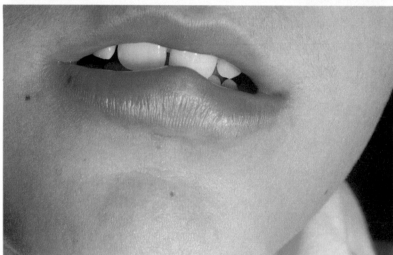

PLEXIFORM NEUROMA. Female; *age* 11 years; *duration* 1 year; lower lip; confirmed by biopsy.

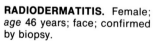**RADIODERMATITIS.** Female; *age* 46 years; face; confirmed by biopsy.

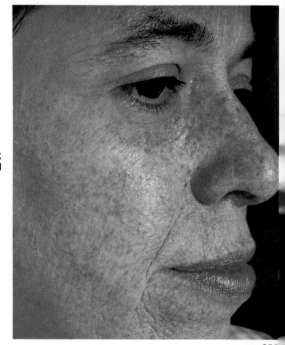

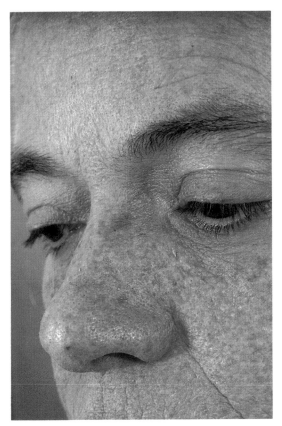

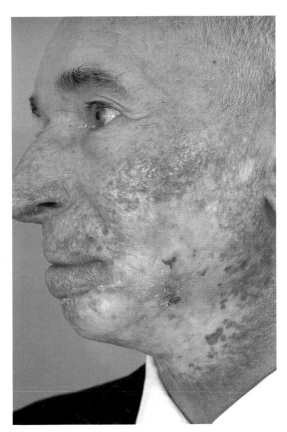

RADIODERMATITIS. Female; *age* 46 years; face. (Same patient as in previous photograph.)

RADIODERMATITIS. Male; *age* 65 years; face; confirmed by biopsy.

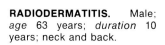

RADIODERMATITIS. Male; *age* 63 years; *duration* 10 years; neck and back.

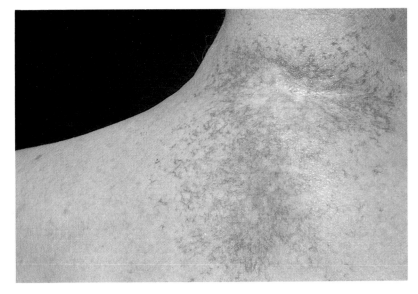

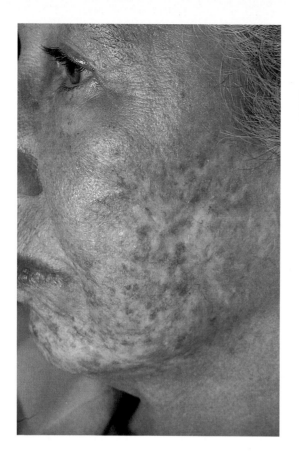

RADIODERMATITIS. Female; *age* 67 years; face; confirmed by biopsy.

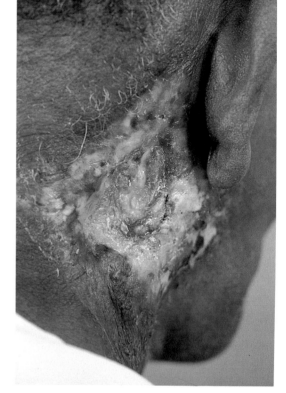

RADIODERMATITIS, WITH ULCERATION. Male; *age* 66 years; *duration* 2 years; neck; confirmed by biopsy.

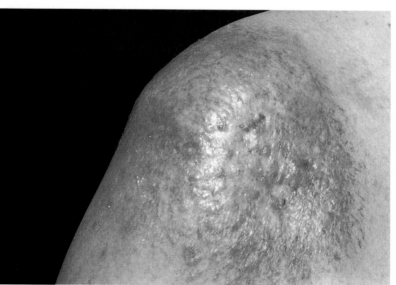

RADIODERMATITIS. Male; *age* 61 years; shoulder; confirmed by biopsy.

RADIODERMATITIS. Male; *age* 60 years; *duration* 9 years; shoulder; confirmed by biopsy.

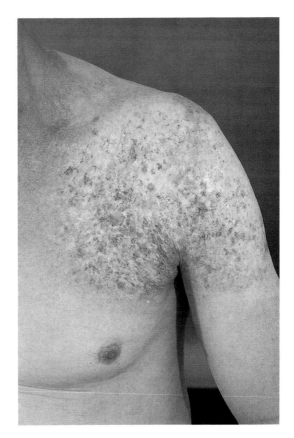

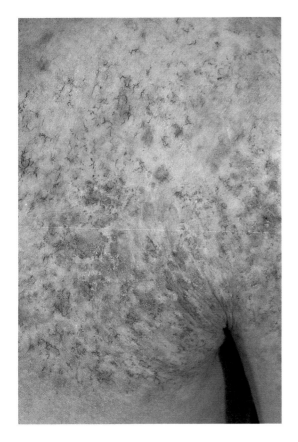

RADIODERMATITIS. Male; *age* 60 years; *duration* 9 years; shoulder; confirmed by biopsy. (Same patient as in previous photograph.)

RADIODERMATITIS. Female; *age* 68 years; chest and axilla.

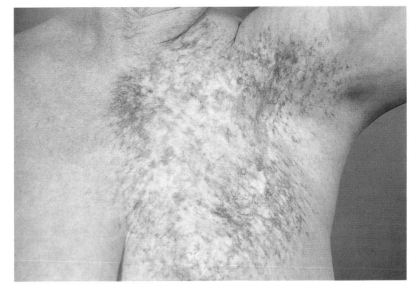

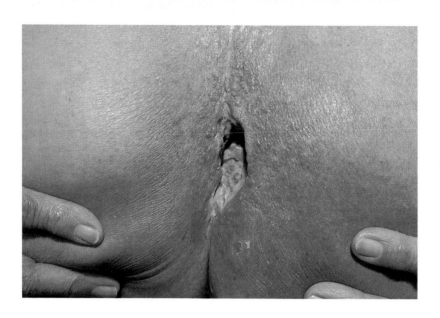

RADIODERMATITIS WITH ULCERATION. Female; *age* 67 years; inter gluteal area; confirmed by biopsy.

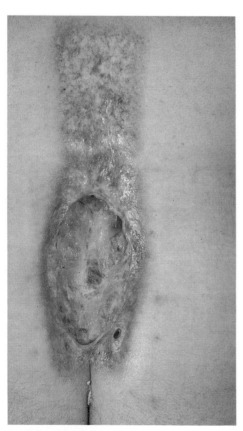

RADIODERMATITIS WITH ULCERATION. Male; *age* 40 years; *duration* 9 years; lumbosacral area; confirmed by biopsy.

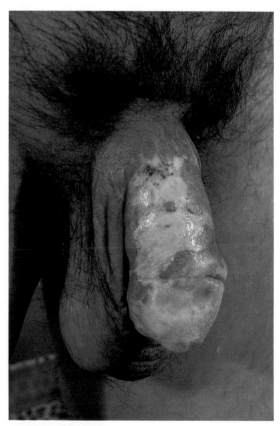

RADIODERMATITIS. Male; *age* 36 years; *duration* 11 years; penis; confirmed by biopsy.

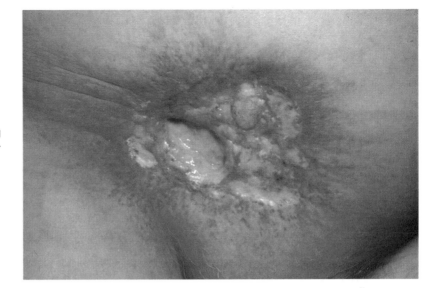

RADIODERMATITIS, WITH ULCERATION. Female; suprapubic area.

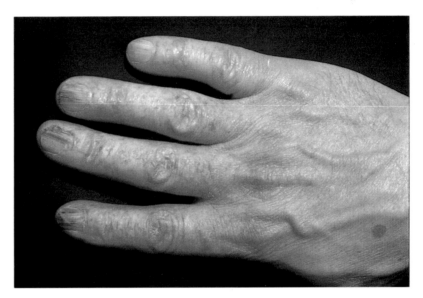

RADIODERMATITIS WITH ONYCHODYSTROPHY. Male; *age* 60 years; *duration* 4 years; fingers; confirmed by biopsy.

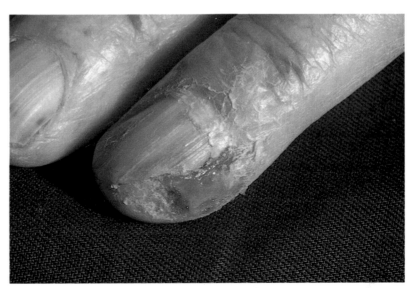

RADIODERMATITIS. Male; *age* 60 years; *duration* 5 years; finger; confirmed by biopsy.

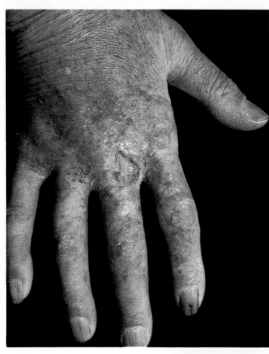

RADIODERMATITIS. Male; *age* 74 years; *duration* 45 years; hand.

RETICULOHISTIOCYTOSIS, MULTICENTRIC. Female; *age* 42 years; *duration* 8 years; neck; confirmed by biopsy.

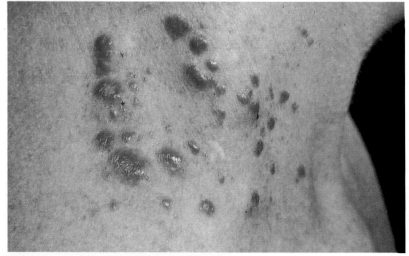

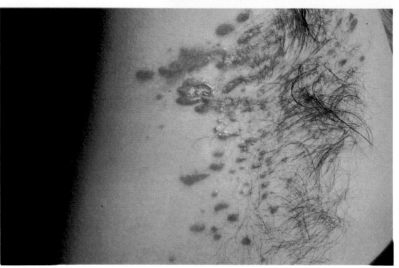

RETICULOHISTIOCYTOSIS, MULTICENTRIC. Female; age 42 years; *duration* 8 years; axilla; confirmed by biopsy. (Same patient as in previous photograph.)

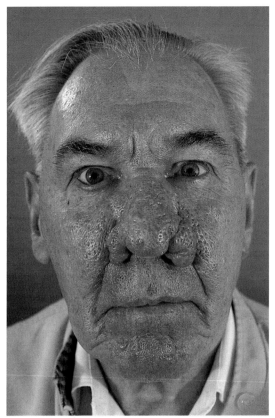

RHINOPHYMA. Male; *age* 68 years; *duration* 15 years; nose.

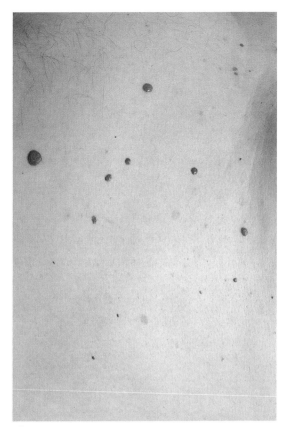

RUBY (SENILE) ANGIOMAS. Male; *age* 73 years; trunk.

RUBY (SENILE) ANGIOMA. Male; chest.

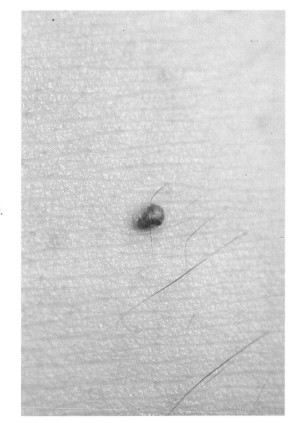

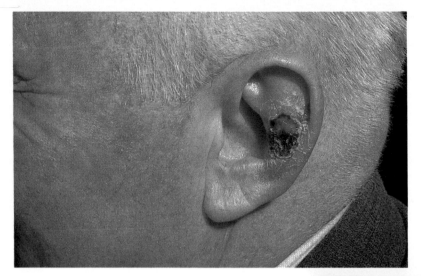

SARCOMA (UNDIFFERENTI-ATED). Male; *age* 66 years; *duration* 3 months; ear; confirmed by biopsy.

SARCOMA (ALVEOLAR RHABDOMYOSARCOMA). Male; *age* 16 years; *duration* 2 months; foot; confirmed by biopsy.

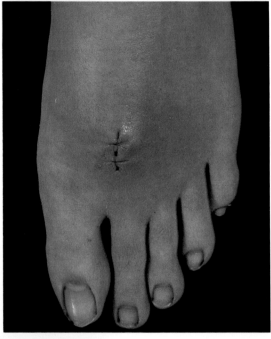

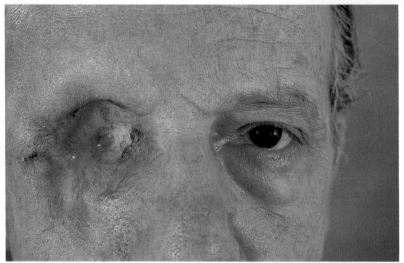

SARCOMA (UNDIFFERENTI-ATED). Male; *age* 64 years; orbital area; confirmed by biopsy.

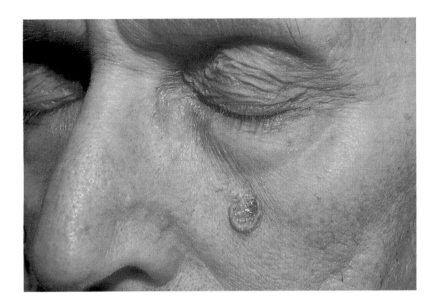

SEBACEOUS GLAND ADEN-OMA. Male; *age* 88 years; cheek; confirmed by biopsy.

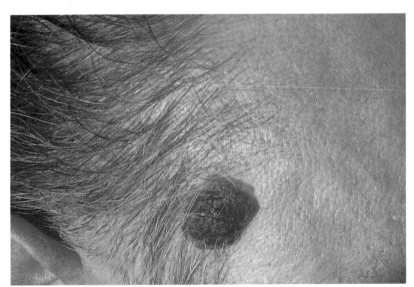

SEBORRHEIC KERATOSIS. Male; *age* 53 years; *duration* 7 years; temple; confirmed by biopsy.

SEBORRHEIC KERATOSIS. Male; *age* 84 years; *duration* 2 years; forehead.

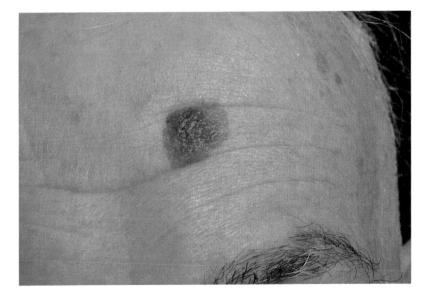

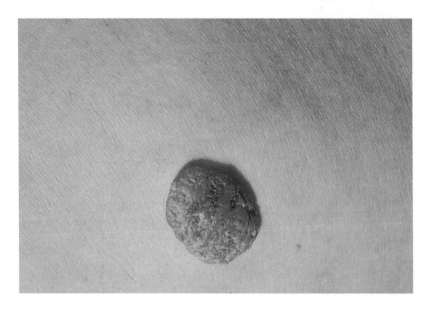

SEBORRHEIC KERATOSIS.
Male; *age* 62 years; *duration* 20 years; back; confirmed by biopsy.

SEBORRHEIC KERATOSIS.
Male; *age* 71 years; *duration* 8 years; cheek; confirmed by biopsy.

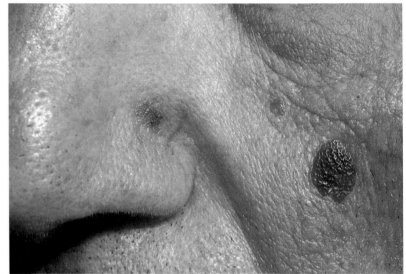

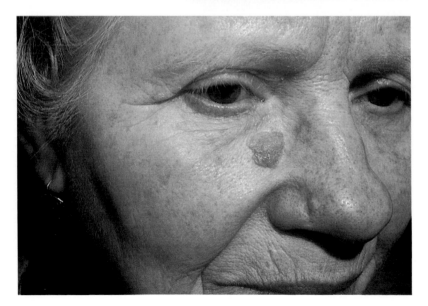

SEBORRHEIC KERATOSIS.
Female; *age* 67 years; *duration* 10 years; cheek; confirmed by biopsy.

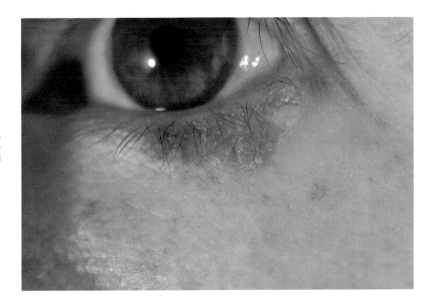

SEBORRHEIC KERATOSIS.
Female; *age* 49 years; *duration* 5 years; eyelid; confirmed by biopsy.

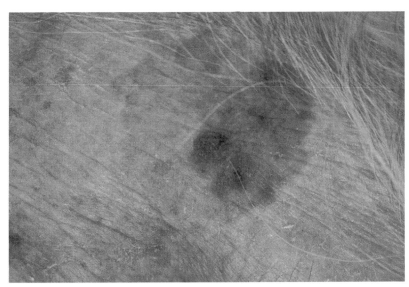

SEBORRHEIC KERATOSIS.
Female; *age* 60 years; temple; confirmed by biopsy.

SEBORRHEIC KERATOSIS.
Female; *age* 52 years; *duration* 25 years; cheek; confirmed by biopsy.

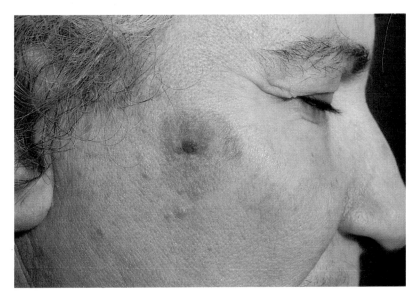

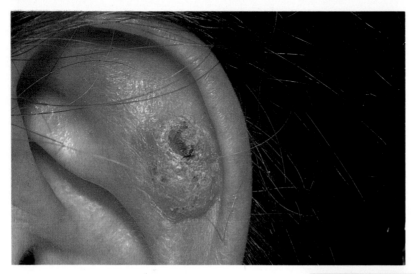

SEBORRHEIC KERATOSIS.
Female; *age* 56 years; *duration* 5–7 months; ear; confirmed by biopsy.

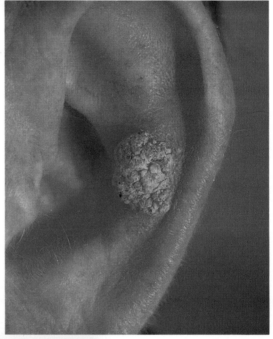

SEBORRHEIC KERATOSIS.
Male; *age* 64 years; *duration* 1 year; ear; confirmed by biopsy.

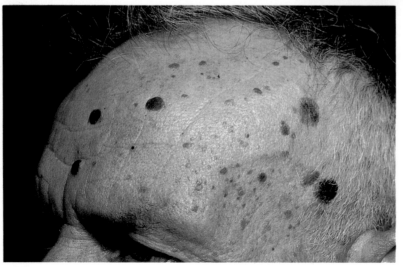

SEBORRHEIC KERATOSES.
Male; *age* 68 years; forehead and temple; confirmed by biopsy.

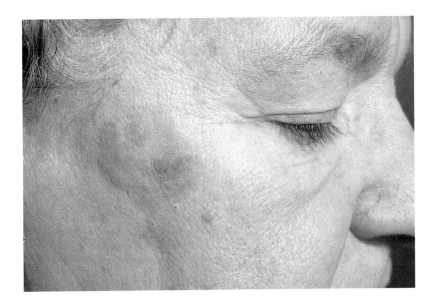

SEBORRHEIC KERATOSIS.
Female; *age* 66 years; *duration* 2 years; cheek; confirmed by biopsy.

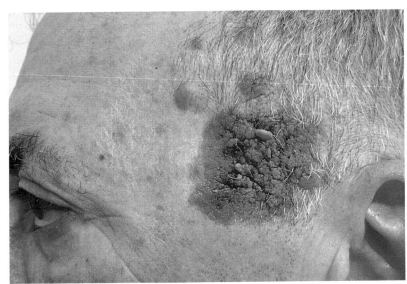

SEBORRHEIC KERATOSIS.
Male; *age* 66 years; *duration* 2 years; temple; confirmed by biopsy.

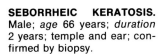

SEBORRHEIC KERATOSIS.
Male; *age* 66 years; *duration* 2 years; temple and ear; confirmed by biopsy.

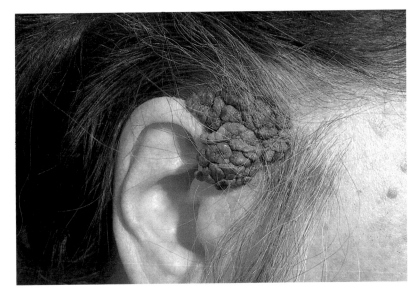

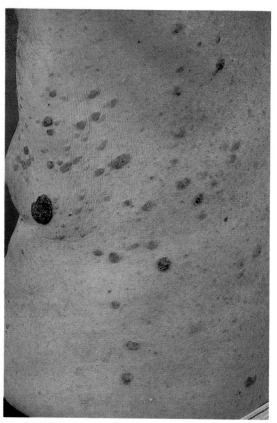

SEBORRHEIC KERATOSES. Male; *age* 74 years; trunk; confirmed by biopsy.

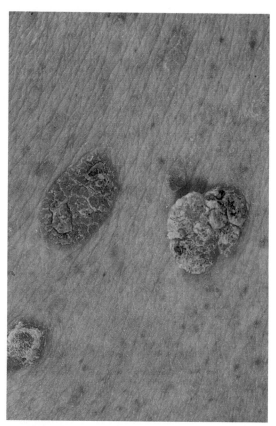

SEBORRHEIC KERATOSES. Male; *age* 74 years; trunk. (Same patient as in previous photograph.)

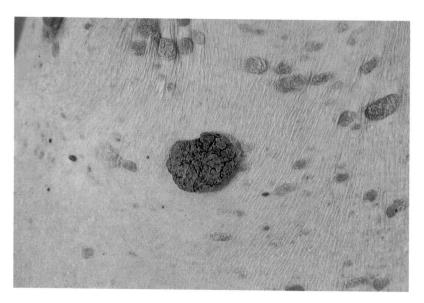

SEBORRHEIC KERATOSES. Male; *age* 74 years; trunk; confirmed by biopsy. (Same patient as in previous photograph.)

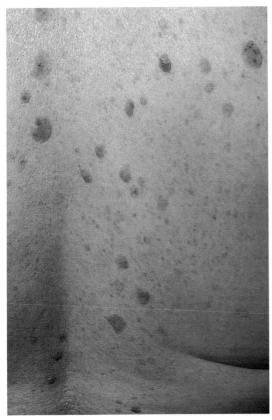

SEBORRHEIC KERATOSES. Male; *age* 69 years; trunk; confirmed by biopsy.

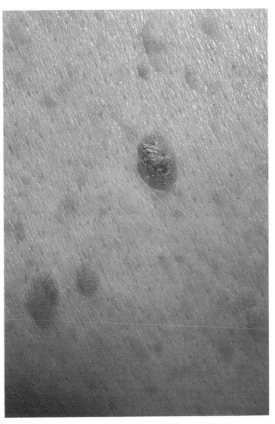

SEBORRHEIC KERATOSES. Male; *age* 69 years; trunk; confirmed by biopsy.

SEBORRHEIC KERATOSIS. Male; *age* 44 years; breast; confirmed by biopsy.

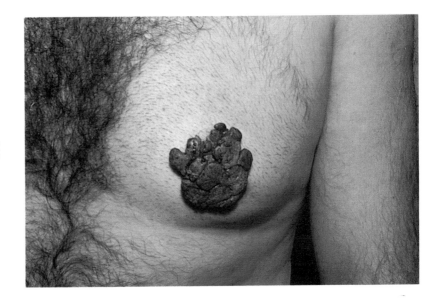

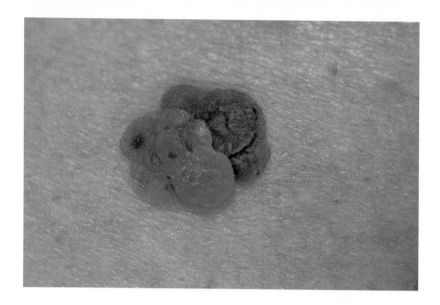

SEBORRHEIC KERATOSIS.
Female; *age* 62 years; back;
confirmed by biopsy.

SEBORRHEIC KERATOSIS.
Male; *age* 65 years; *duration*
10 years; thigh; confirmed by
biopsy.

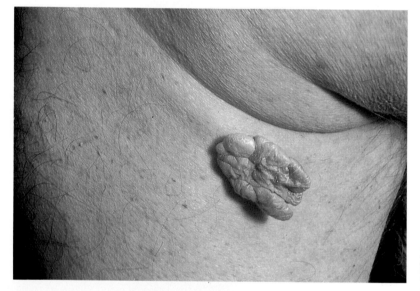

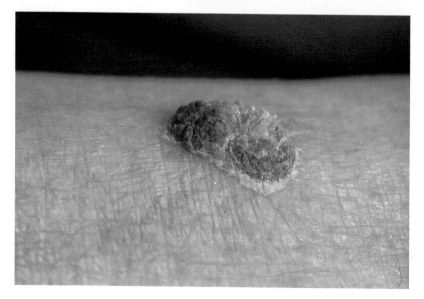

SEBORRHEIC KERATOSIS.
Female; *age* 72 years; calf;
confirmed by biopsy.

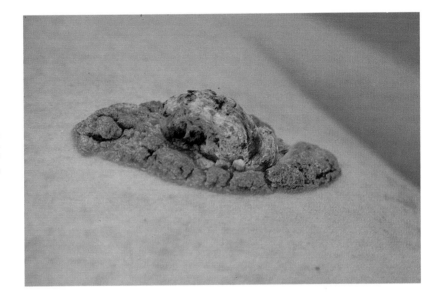

SEBORRHEIC KERATOSIS. (WITH CUTANEOUS HORN). Male; *age* 64 years; *duration* 20 years; confirmed by biopsy.

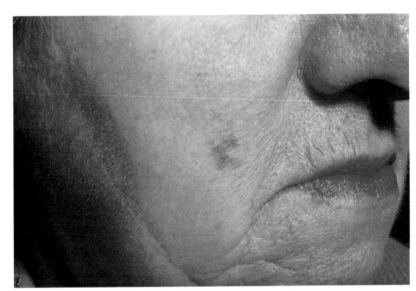

SOLAR LENTIGO. Female; *age* 62 years; *duration* 10 years; cheek; confirmed by biopsy.

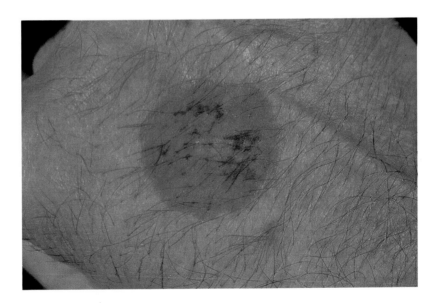

SOLAR LENTIGO. Male; 75 years; *duration* 10 years; hand.

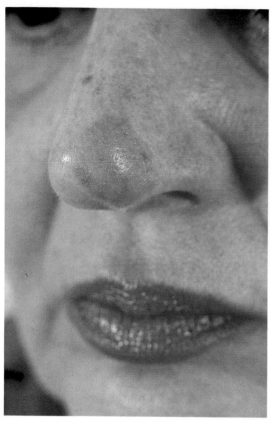

SOLAR LENTIGO. Female; nose.

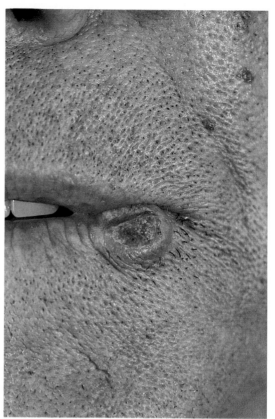

SQUAMOUS-CELL CARCINOMA. Male; *age* 60 years; *duration* 18 years; lower lip; confirmed by biopsy.

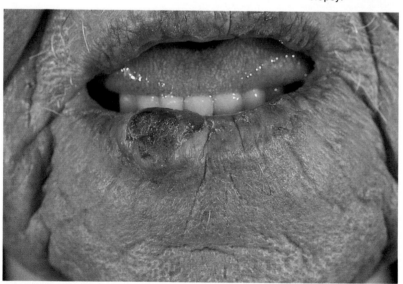

SQUAMOUS-CELL CARCI-NOMA. Female; *age* 80 years; *duration* 6 months; lower lip; confirmed by biopsy.

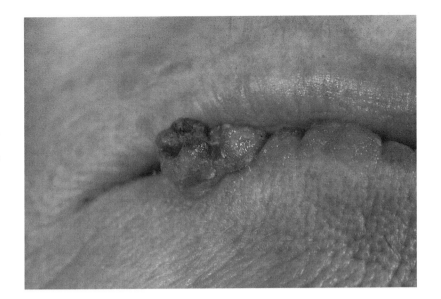

SQUAMOUS-CELL CARCI-NOMA. Female; *age* 59 years; *duration* 1 year; lower lip; confirmed by biopsy.

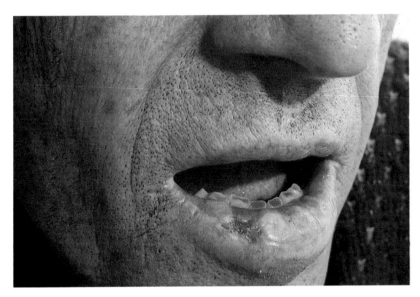

SQUAMOUS-CELL CARCI-NOMA. Male; *age* 59 years; *duration* 9 months; lip; confirmed by biopsy.

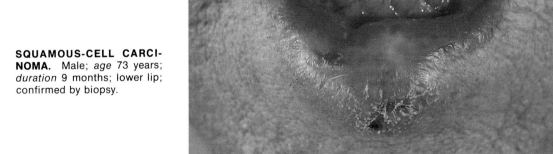

SQUAMOUS-CELL CARCI-NOMA. Male; *age* 73 years; *duration* 9 months; lower lip; confirmed by biopsy.

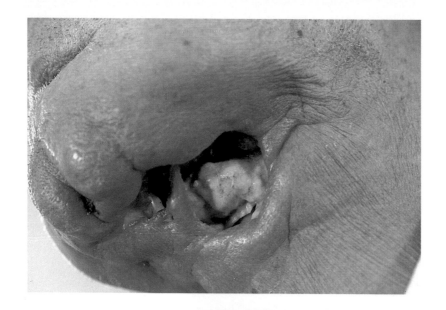

SQUAMOUS-CELL CARCI-NOMA (METASTATIC FROM LIP). Male; *age* 74 years; *duration* 9 months; submental area; confirmed by biopsy.

SQUAMOUS-CELL CARCI-NOMA. Male; lower lip.

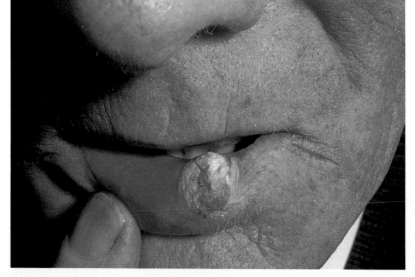

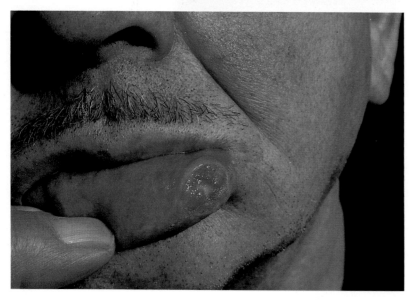

SQUAMOUS-CELL CARCI-NOMA. Male; *age* 73 years; *duration* 3 months; lower lip; confirmed by biopsy.

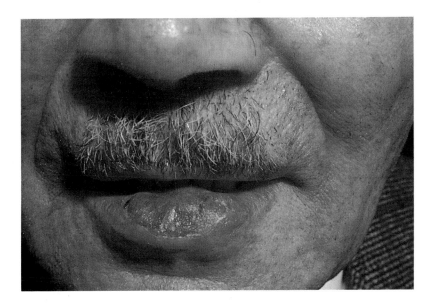

SQUAMOUS-CELL CARCI-NOMA. Male; *age* 77 years; *duration* 3 years; lower lip; confirmed by biopsy.

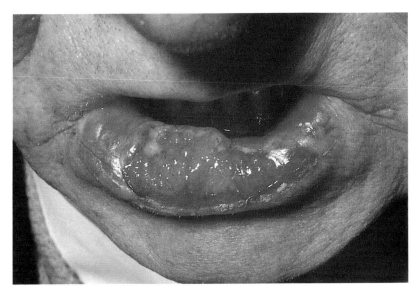

SQUAMOUS-CELL CARCI-NOMA. Male; *age* 60 years; *duration* 3 years; lower lip; confirmed by biopsy.

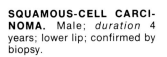

SQUAMOUS-CELL CARCI-NOMA. Male; *duration* 4 years; lower lip; confirmed by biopsy.

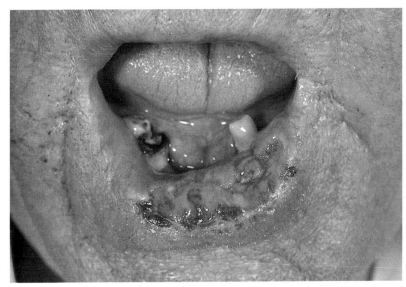

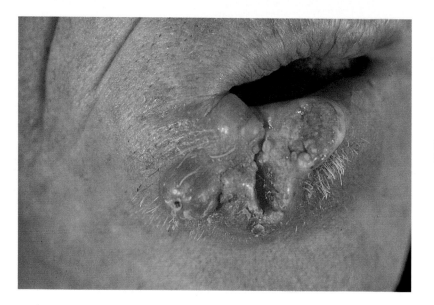

SQUAMOUS-CELL CARCI-NOMA. Male; lower lip.

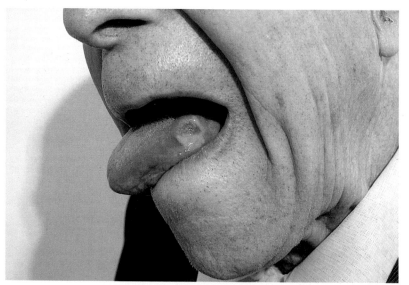

SQUAMOUS-CELL CARCI-NOMA. Male; *age* 77 years; *duration* 2 years; tongue; con-firmed by biopsy.

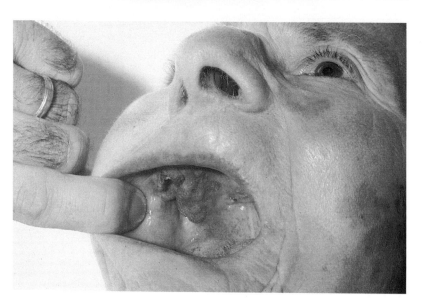

SQUAMOUS-CELL CARCI-NOMA. Female; *age* 70 years; *duration* 6 months; palate; confirmed by biopsy.

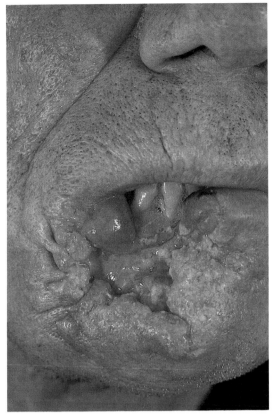

SQUAMOUS-CELL CARCINOMA. Male; *age* 59 years; lower lip; confirmed by biopsy.

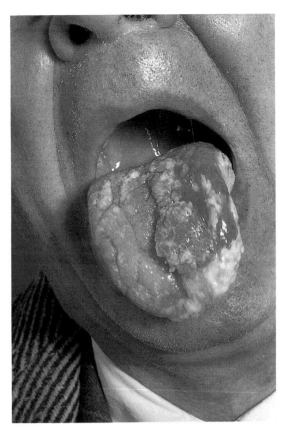

SQUAMOUS-CELL CARCINOMA. Male; tongue.

SQUAMOUS-CELL CARCINOMA (IN RADIODERMA-TITIS). Male; *age* 57 years; scalp; confirmed by biopsy.

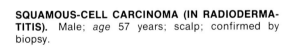

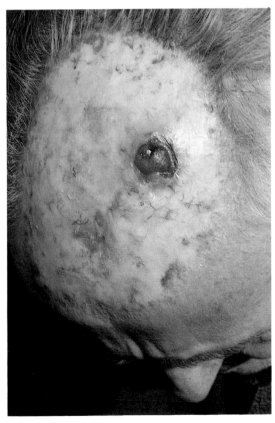

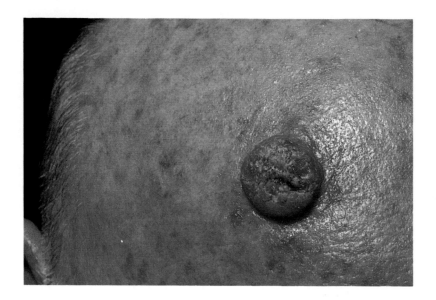

**SQUAMOUS-CELL CARCI-
NOMA.** Male; *age* 60 years;
duration 3 months; forehead;
confirmed by biopsy.

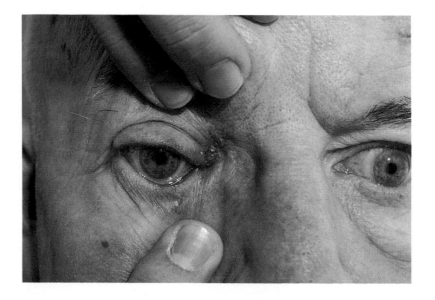

**SQUAMOUS-CELL CARCI-
NOMA.** Male; *age* 73 years;
duration 6 months; inner canthal area; confirmed by biopsy.

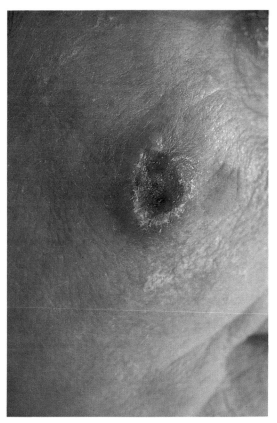

SQUAMOUS-CELL CARCINOMA. Female; *age* 67 years; *duration* 6 months; cheek; confirmed by biopsy.

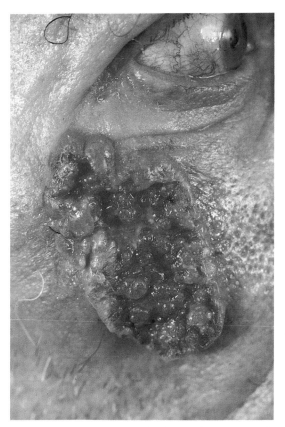

SQUAMOUS-CELL CARCINOMA. Male; *age* 67 years; *duration* 2 months; cheek; confirmed by biopsy.

SQUAMOUS-CELL CARCI-NOMA. Male; *age* 85 years; *duration* 1 year; temple; confirmed by biopsy.

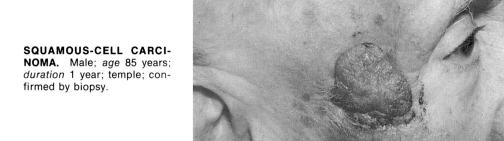

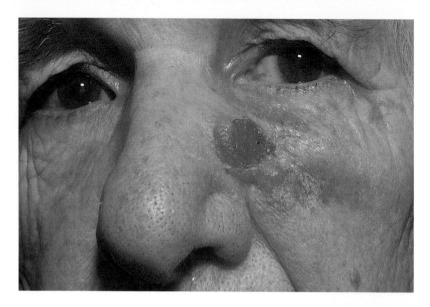

SQUAMOUS-CELL CARCI-NOMA. Female; *age* 80 years; nose; confirmed by biopsy.

SQUAMOUS-CELL CARCI-NOMA. Male; *age* 74 years; *duration* 3 years; paranasal area; confirmed by biopsy.

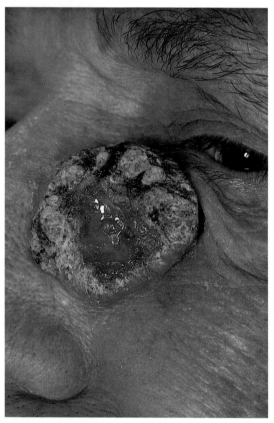

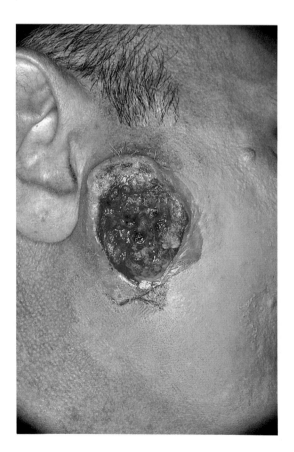

SQUAMOUS-CELL CARCI-NOMA. Male; *age* 56 years; *duration* 2 years; cheek; con-firmed by biopsy.

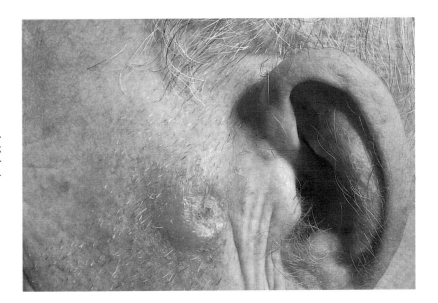

SQUAMOUS-CELL CARCI-NOMA. Male; *age* 69 years; *duration* 3 months; preauricular area; confirmed by biopsy.

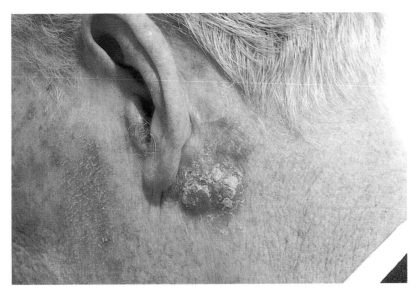

SQUAMOUS-CELL CARCI-NOMA. Male; *age* 72 years; *duration* 6 months; retroauricular area; confirmed by biopsy.

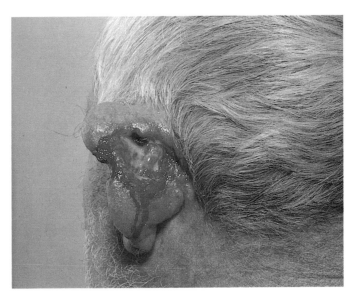

SQUAMOUS-CELL CARCI-NOMA. Male; *age* 86 years; *duration* 6 months; ear; confirmed by biopsy.

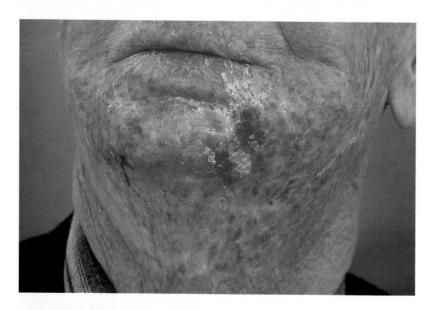

SQUAMOUS-CELL CARCINOMA (IN RADIODERMATITIS). Male; *age* 67 years; *duration* 3 months; chin; confirmed by biopsy.

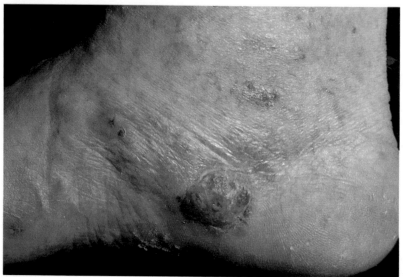

SQUAMOUS-CELL CARCINOMA. Male; *age* 64 years; *duration* 1 year; foot; confirmed by biopsy.

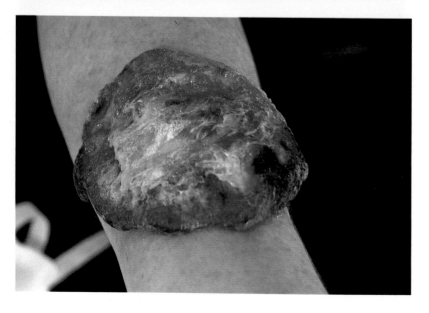

SQUAMOUS-CELL CARCINOMA. Female; *age* 54 years; *duration* 1 year; forearm; confirmed by biopsy.

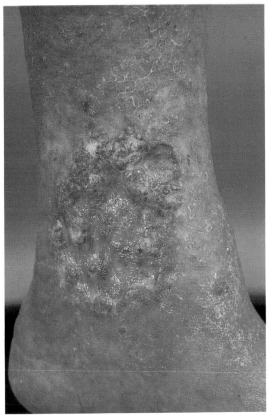

SQUAMOUS-CELL CARCINOMA. Female; *age* 66 years; *duration* 5 years; leg; confirmed by biopsy.

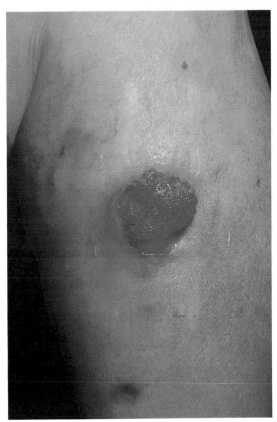

SQUAMOUS-CELL CARCINOMA. Female; *age* 74 years; *duration* 16 months; leg; confirmed by biopsy.

SQUAMOUS-CELL CARCINOMA (IN BURN SCAR).
Female; *age* 40 years; leg; confirmed by biopsy.

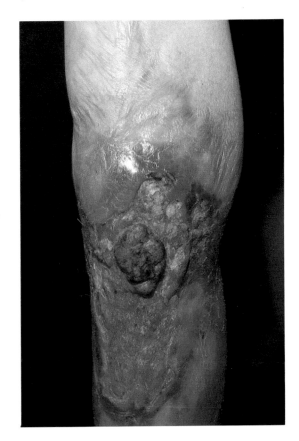

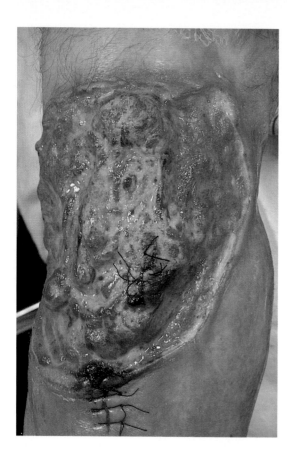

SQUAMOUS-CELL CARCI-NOMA. Male; *age* 63 years; leg; confirmed by biopsy.

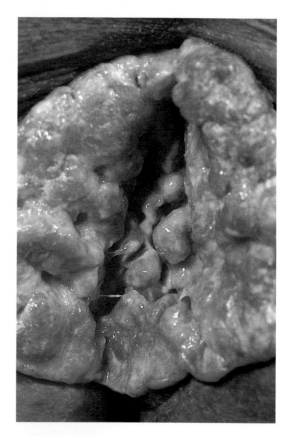

SQUAMOUS-CELL CARCI-NOMA. Female; *age* 60 years; *duration* 3 months; anal area; confirmed by biopsy.

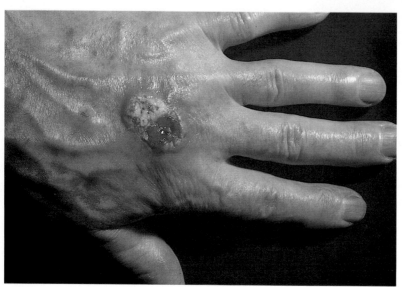

SQUAMOUS-CELL CARCI-NOMA. Male; *age* 68 years; *duration* 5 years; hand; confirmed by biopsy.

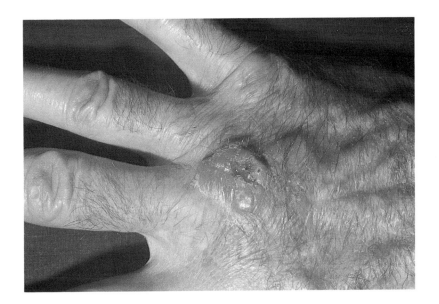

SQUAMOUS-CELL CARCI-NOMA. Male; hand.

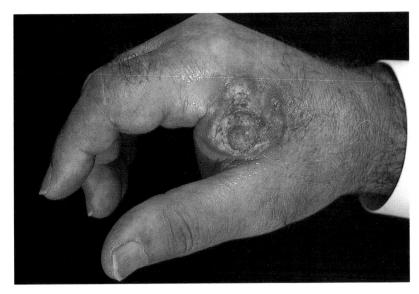

SQUAMOUS-CELL CARCI-NOMA. Male; *age* 57 years; *duration* 4 years; hand; confirmed by biopsy.

SQUAMOUS-CELL CARCI-NOMA. Female; *age* 80 years; *duration* 6 months; interdigital web; confirmed by biopsy.

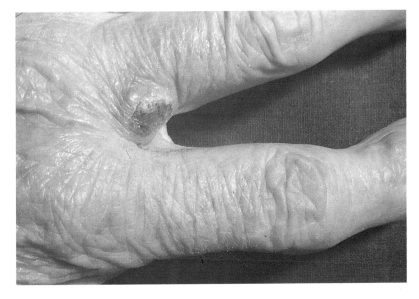

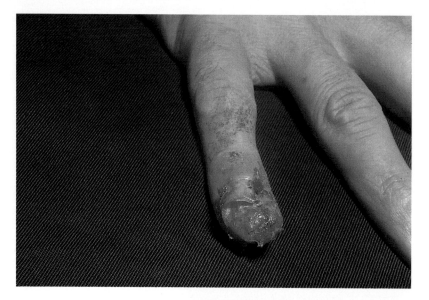

**SQUAMOUS-CELL CARCI-
NOMA.** Female; *age* 63 years;
duration 20 months; finger;
confirmed by biopsy.

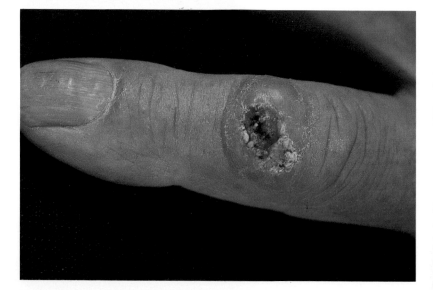

**SQUAMOUS-CELL CARCI-
NOMA.** Male; *age* 69 years;
finger; confirmed by biopsy.

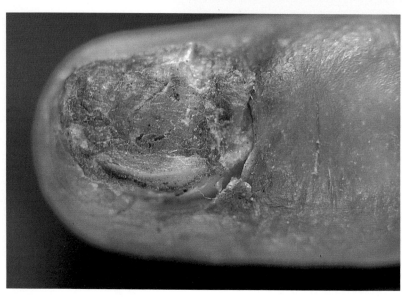

**SQUAMOUS-CELL CARCI-
NOMA.** Male; *age* 42 years;
finger; confirmed by biopsy.

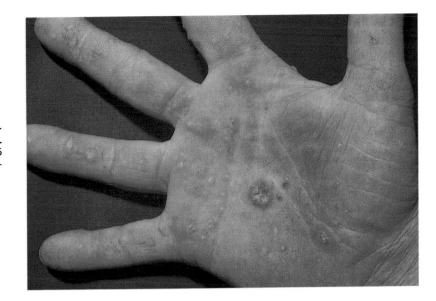

SQUAMOUS-CELL CARCI-NOMA (AND ARSENICAL KERATOSES). Male; *age* 45 years; palm; confirmed by biopsy.

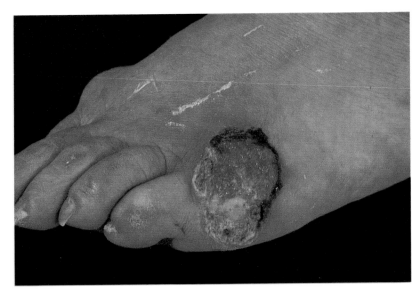

SQUAMOUS-CELL CARCI-NOMA. Male; *age* 70 years; *duration* 2 years; foot; confirmed by biopsy.

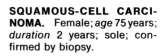

SQUAMOUS-CELL CARCI-NOMA. Female; *age* 75 years; *duration* 2 years; sole; confirmed by biopsy.

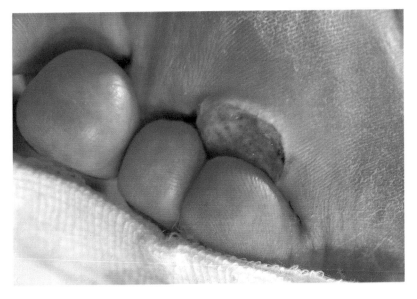

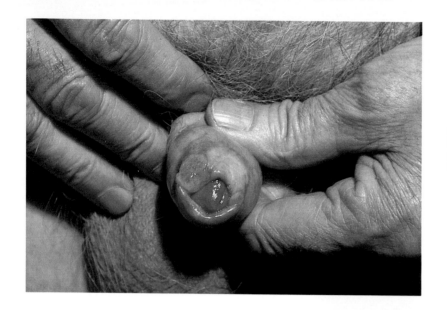

SQUAMOUS-CELL CARCI-NOMA. Male; *age* 74 years; *duration* 6 months; penis; confirmed by biopsy.

SQUAMOUS-CELL CARCI-NOMA. Male; *age* 79 years; *duration* 16 months; penis; confirmed by biopsy.

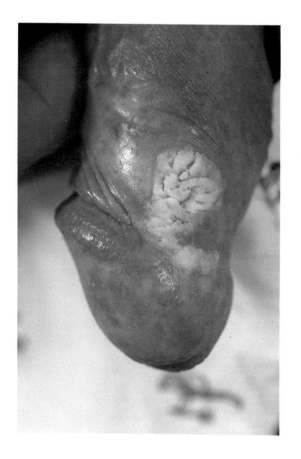

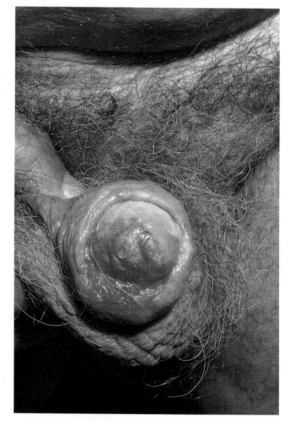

SQUAMOUS-CELL CARCI-NOMA. Male; *age* 70 years; *duration* 3 months; penis; confirmed by biopsy.

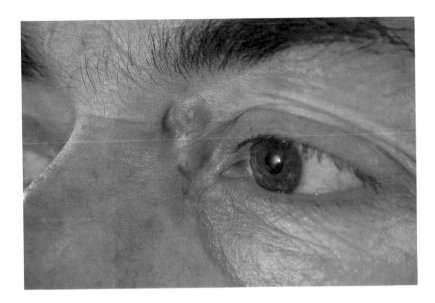

SWEAT GLAND ADENOMA.
Male; *age* 47 years; *duration* 32 years; inner canthal area; confirmed by biopsy.

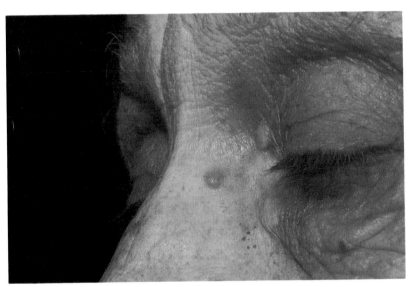

SWEAT GLAND ADENOMA.
Female; *age* 71 years; *duration* 1 month; nose; confirmed by biopsy.

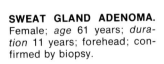

SWEAT GLAND ADENOMA.
Female; *age* 61 years; *duration* 11 years; forehead; confirmed by biopsy.

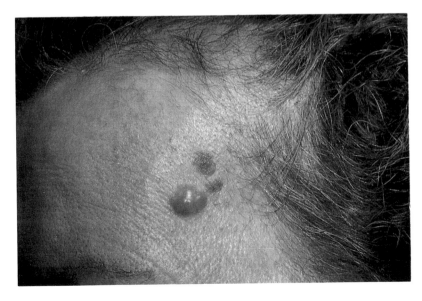

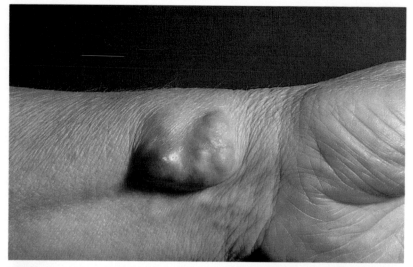

SWEAT GLAND ADENOMA.
Female; *age* 70 years; *duration* 56 years; wrist; confirmed by biopsy.

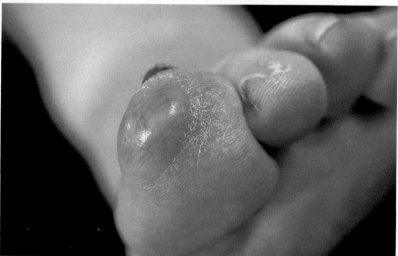

SWEAT GLAND ADENOMA.
Female; *age* 68 years; *duration* 7 years; toe; confirmed by biopsy.

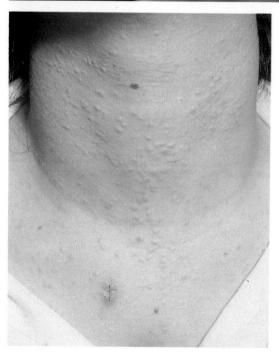

SYRINGOMAS. Female; *age* 22 years; *duration* 9 years; neck and chest; confirmed by biopsy.

SYRINGOMAS. Female; *age* 22 years; *duration* 9 years; eyelids; confirmed by biopsy. (Same patient as in previous photograph.)

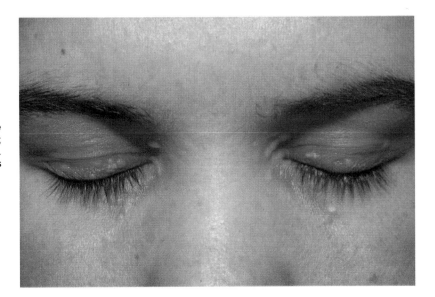

SYRINGOMAS. Female; *age* 53 years; *duration* 20 years; eyelid; confirmed by biopsy.

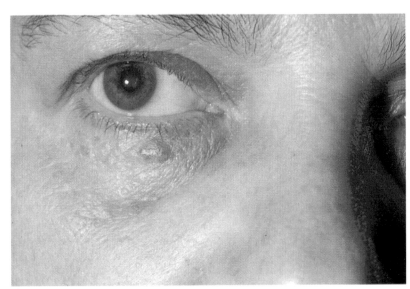

SYRINGOMAS. Male; *age* 22 years; *duration* 7 years; eyelids; confirmed by biopsy.

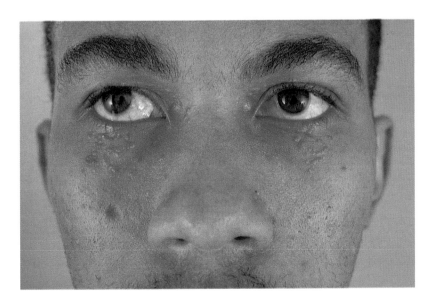

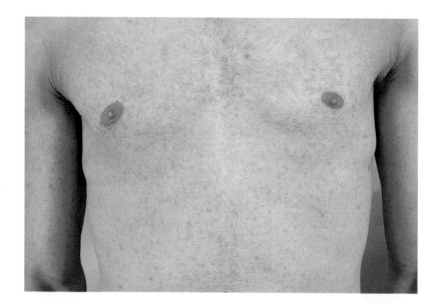

SYRINGOMAS. Male; *age* 22 years; *duration* 7 years; trunk; confirmed by biopsy. (Same patient as in previous photograph.)

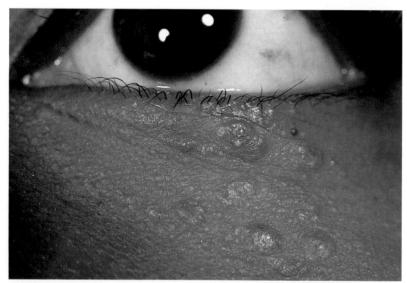

SYRINGOMA. Female; *age* 19 years; *duration* 3 years; eyelid; confirmed by biopsy.

SYRINGOMA. Male; *age* 25 years; *duration* 21 years; neck; confirmed by biopsy.

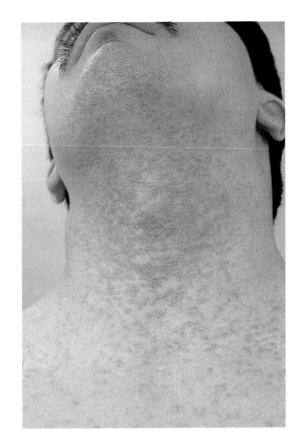

SYRINGOMAS. Male; *age* 25 years; *duration* 21 years; neck and chest; confirmed by biopsy. (Same patient as in previous photograph.)

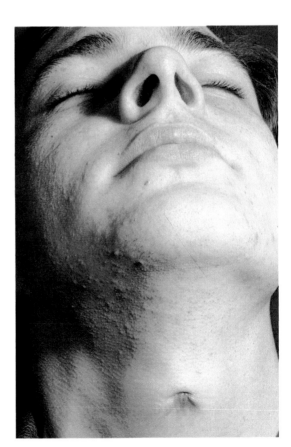

THYROGLOSSAL DUCT CYST. Male; neck.

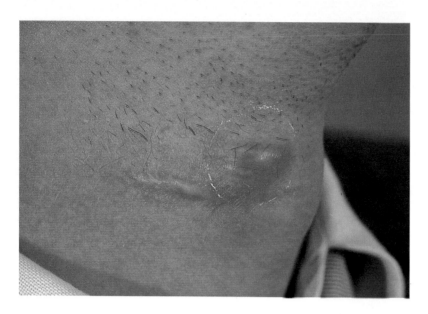

THYROGLOSSAL DUCT CYST. Male; *age* 21 years; neck; confirmed by biopsy.

TRICHOEPITHELIOMAS. Female; face.

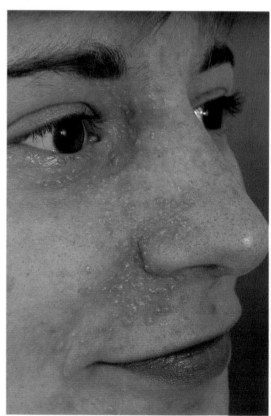

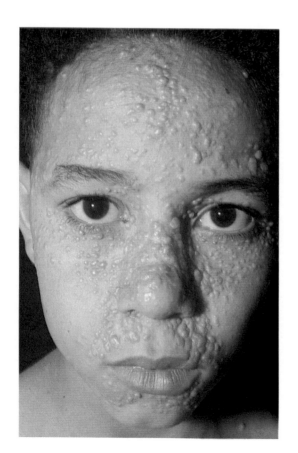

TRICHOEPITHELIOMAS. Male; face.

TRICHOEPITHELIOMAS.
Male; *age* 21 years; face; confirmed by biopsy.

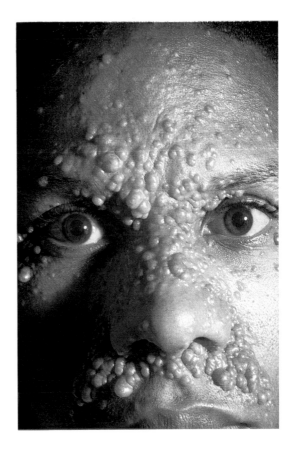

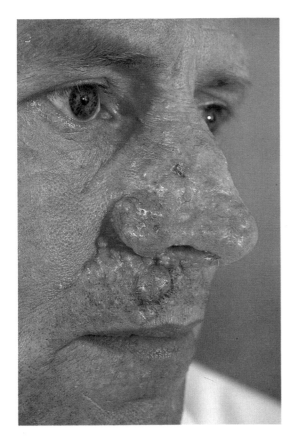

TRICHOEPITHELIOMAS.
Male; *age* 46 years; *duration* 20 years; face; confirmed by biopsy.

TRICHOEPITHELIOMAS.
Male; *age* 42 years; *duration* 20 years; face; confirmed by biopsy.

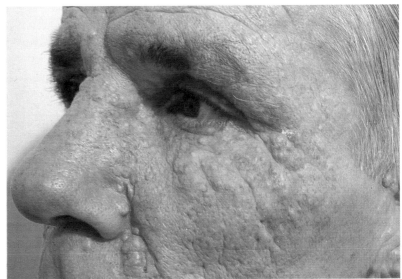

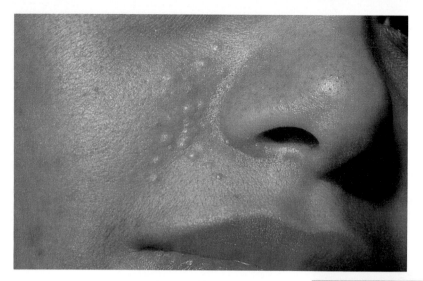

TRICHOEPITHELIOMAS. Female; *age* 19 years; *duration* 7 years; cheek; confirmed by biopsy.

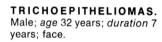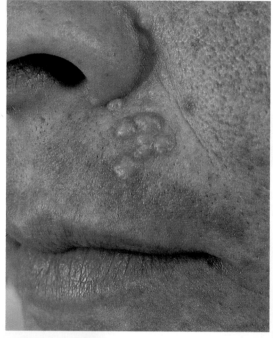

TRICHOEPITHELIOMAS. Male; *age* 32 years; *duration* 7 years; face.

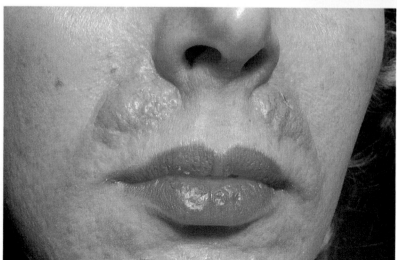

TRICHOEPITHELIOMAS. Female; upper lip.

URTICARIA PIGMENTOSA.
Face and trunk.

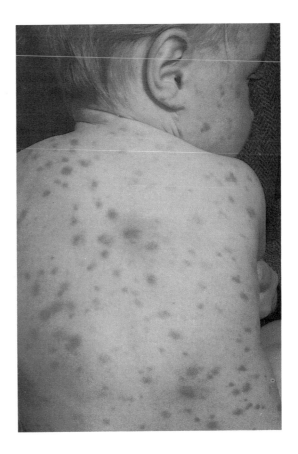

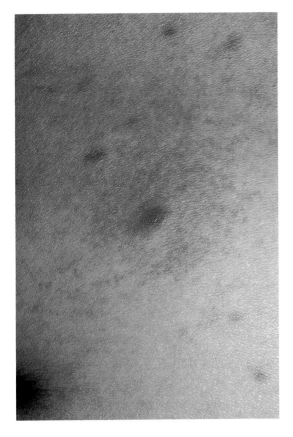

URTICARIA PIGMENTOSA.
Female; *age* 27 years; *duration* 5 years; trunk; confirmed by biopsy.

URTICARIA PIGMENTOSA.
Trunk.

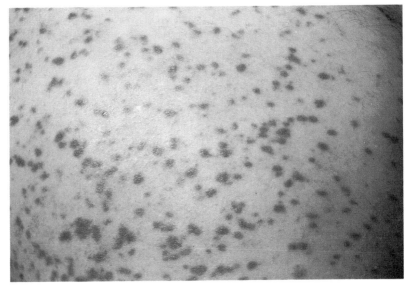

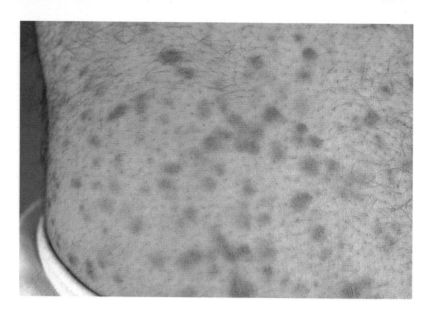

URTICARIA PIGMENTOSA.
Male; *age* 31 years; *duration* 18 years; trunk.

URTICARIA PIGMENTOSA.
Male; *age* 31 years; *duration* 18 years; trunk and arm. (Same patient as in previous photograph.)

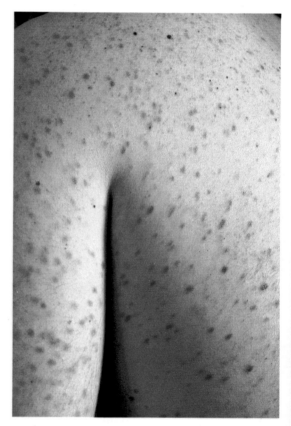

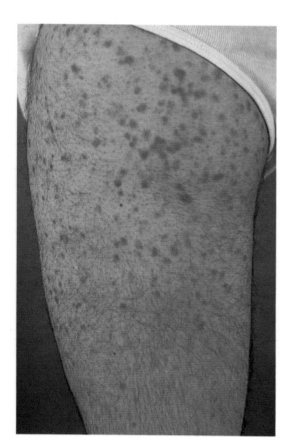

URTICARIA PIGMENTOSA.
Male; *age* 31 years; *duration* 18 years; generalized. (Same patient as in previous photograph.)

URTICARIA PIGMENTOSA.
Female; trunk.

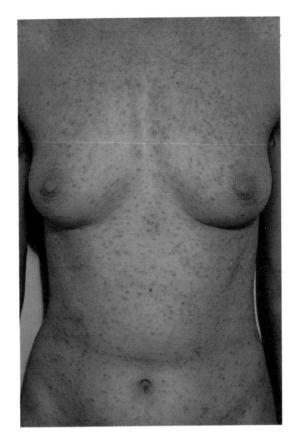

URTICARIA PIGMENTOSA.
Trunk and thigh.

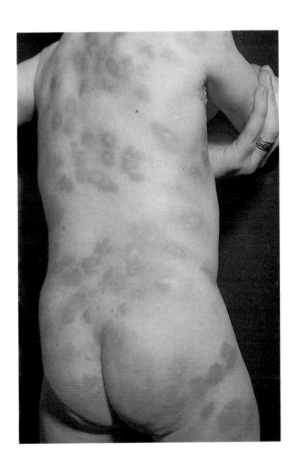

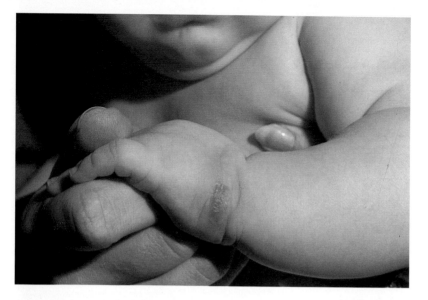

URTICARIA PIGMENTOSA.
Female; *age* 5 months; *duration* 4 months; hand.

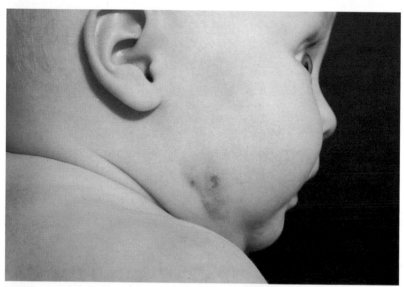

URTICARIA PIGMENTOSA.
Female; *age* 5 months; *duration* 4 months; face. (Same patient as in previous photograph.)

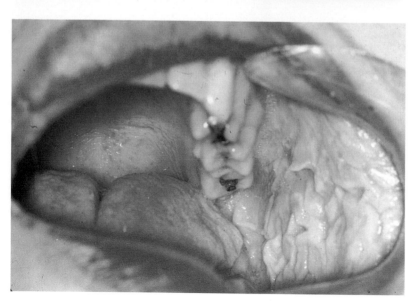

WHITE SPONGE NEVUS.
Buccal mucosa.

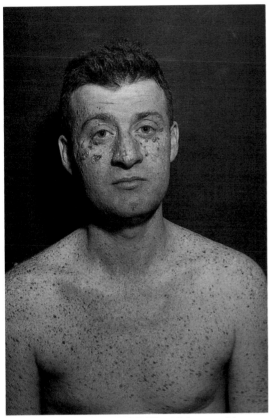

XERODERMA PIGMENTOSUM. Male; *age* 44 years; *duration* 30 years; face and trunk; confirmed by biopsy.

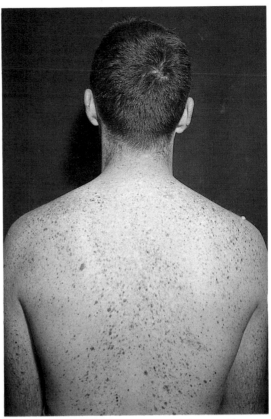

XERODERMA PIGMENTOSUM. Male; *age* 44 years; *duration* 30 years; back; confirmed by biopsy. (Same patient as in previous photograph.)

XERODERMA PIGMENTO-SUM. Male; *age* 54 years; *duration* 40 years; face; confirmed by biopsy. (Same patient as in previous photograph.)

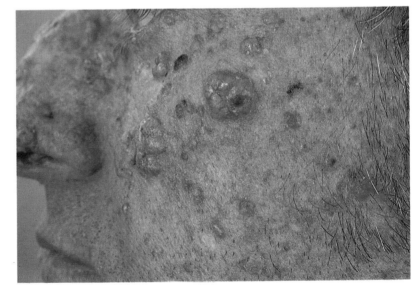

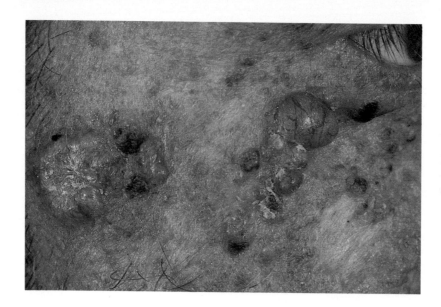

XERODERMA PIGMENTO-SUM. Male; *age* 54 years; *duration* 40 years; face; confirmed by biopsy. (Same patient as in previous photograph.)

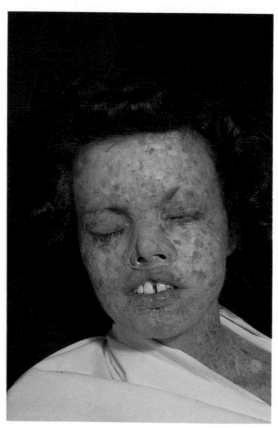

XERODERMA PIGMENTOSUM. Female; *age* 17 years; *duration* since birth; face and neck.

INDEX